# The Social Organization of Best Practice

Fiona Webster

# The Social Organization of Best Practice

An Institutional Ethnography of Physicians' Work

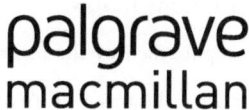

Fiona Webster
Arthur Labatt Family School of Nursing
Western University
London, ON, Canada

ISBN 978-3-030-43164-8      ISBN 978-3-030-43165-5   (eBook)
https://doi.org/10.1007/978-3-030-43165-5

This Palgrave Macmillan imprint is published by the registered company Springer Nature Switzerland AG.
The registered company address is: Gewerbestrasse 11, 6330 Cham, Switzerland

# FOREWORD

This is a remarkable book. It opens up a whole new terrain of exploration and discovery in the health care field that, so far as I know, has never been attempted before. Though Fiona Webster does not give a detailed account here, her dissertation, on which this draws, gathered together the research literature establishing 'best practices' for the treatment of thrombolytic strokes. The venture of discovery she undertook and recounts in this book found and made visible 'best practices' as they are taken up in actual local situations of medical practice in the Canadian province of Ontario.

This is valuable work, with implications way beyond those for the particular case of therapy for thrombolytic strokes. Its significance is not only in what we learn about how 'best practice' recommendations may be grounded in assumptions about the availability of specialized skills and relevant technology which are not always present in the actual local situations of delivery work. What Webster brings into view is the significance of the actual local organization of professional work in realizing as a local reality the abstract generalizations of medical research.

Webster's research deploys a sociology known as 'institutional ethnography'. It is distinctive in enabling exploration of how the generalized forms of institutional organization such as health care are actually put together as people's local practices. Ethnography as a sociological method is one of observing people's doings. We might think of it as like the work of ethologists such a Jane Goodall observing how wild primates put their lives together. Institutional ethnography, however, has made a big shift by incorporating into its ethnographic practices the replicable texts that organize peoples' doings across different places and at different times. While ethnographic method as observation limits research to the local and particular of observation, institutional ethnography reaches into dimensions of contemporary society extending beyond the local. Complex forms of organizing what people do are mediated by texts that can generalize uses of language, numbers, sound and image across multiple local settings and at different times. What institutional ethnography introduces is the possibility of exploring ethnographically those remarkable forms of organizing contemporary society that are coordinated by material texts—print, film photos, television, electronic, social media, radio, x-rays, CT scans and so on. Recognizing texts as they come into play in people's actual courses of action, coordinating their doings with those of others, makes it possible to extend ethnography beyond the directly observable and into what can be learned from respondents or by observations grounded in the researcher's experience about their text-coordinated actions. In Webster's institutional ethnography, she brings into view how physicians' actual practices are engaged with textual representations of best practices that have been built on research that takes no account of the very different situations of work in which treatment decisions are made.

Webster's research was in the context of a job that involved travelling to different parts of Ontario. She was thus able to talk to doctors working in different types of hospital and in very different regional settings. The medical research resulting in 'best practice' recommendations for thrombolytic strokes was done under highly controlled situations and relied on technology and highly specialized professional skills which cannot be taken for granted in the community hospitals which are the only source of hospital care in parts of Ontario's province and distant from larger cities. Webster's institutional ethnography not only is valuable in opening up the actual work organization presupposed by these 'best practice' recommendations but also promises an ethnographic approach to the workings of health care systems as what people are actually getting done and under what actual conditions. It suggests also a further step of institutional ethnography that would bring into view the overarching organizing by government or corporation as it enters into and shapes local practices where patient care is actually happening. This makes it a valuable contribution to the IE body of knowledge and a highly recommended book for those teaching or working with IE in health care.

Department of Social Justice Education,
OISE, University of Toronto, Toronto, Canada          Dorothy E. Smith

# Acknowledgements

The considerable knowledge and support of several people enabled me to undertake this study. First, I want to thank everyone who was affiliated with the Ontario Stroke Strategy as well as the clinicians, patients and family members who generously shared their stories. In particular, I would like to acknowledge two people, Christina O'Callaghan and Dr Vladimir Hachinski, whose support and expert guidance has been invaluable to my work. Dr. Hachinski supported my work as a sociologist and took the time to thoughtfully explain the clinical world to me with great patience. I had not realized at the time how unique he was in his generosity; he opened many doors that enabled me to conduct this study and also to establish my career as an embedded sociologist working in health care settings.

This study continues the method of inquiry developed by Dorothy Smith. Her mentorship and friendship over many years has been an extraordinary privilege in my life. She has taught me how to think critically, how to demand more of my work and how to find and trust my own voice. This has changed forever the possibilities I am able to imagine for myself. There exists a large international community of institutional ethnography (IE) researchers and I am indebted to many of them at the personal level and to all of them for their superb work in advancing IE scholarship.

Kathleen Rice kindly put the publication of this work into motion by introducing me to the wonderful Mary Al-Sayed, Commissioning

Editor, Sociology and Anthropology at Palgrave Macmillan, and Editorial Assistant Madison Allums. They provided excellent guidance in shepherding this book through to publication. Finally, a special thank you to Stephan Dobson for his invaluable help in editing this book. It would not exist in its current form without his both superb editing skills and deep knowledge of institutional ethnography.

# CONTENTS

# Acronyms and Abbreviations

| | |
|---|---|
| AHA | American Heart Association |
| AHSC | Academic Health Sciences Centre |
| CAEP | Canadian Association of Emergency Room Physicians |
| CIHR | Canadian Institutes for Health Research |
| CSN | Canadian Stroke Network |
| CT | computed tomography |
| DHC | District Health Council |
| DSC | District Stroke Centre |
| EBM | Evidence-based medicine |
| HSFO | Heart and Stroke Foundation of Ontario |
| ICES | Institute for Clinical Evaluative Sciences |
| IE | Institutional ethnography |
| KT | Knowledge translation |
| LHIN | Local Health Integration Network |
| MoA | Memorandum of Agreement |
| MoHLTC | Ministry of Health and Long-Term Care (Ontario) |
| MRI | Magnetic resonance imaging |
| NINDS | National Institute of Neurological Disorders and Stroke |
| NP | Nurse practitioner |
| NPM | New public management |
| OSS | Ontario Stroke Strategy |
| RCTs | Randomized controlled trials |
| RN | Registered nurse |
| RSC | Regional Stroke Centre |
| rt-PA | Thrombolytic therapy |
| SEAC | Stroke Evaluation Advisory Committee |

CHAPTER 1

# Introduction

This book represents a now historical ethnographic account of a particular time in which the Ontario Stroke Strategy (OSS) was being implemented in Ontario, Canada, with the explicit aim of 'improving best practice care across the continuum'.[1] It offers an explication of how the discourses of both evidence-based medicine (EBM) and knowledge translation (KT) were institutionalized in the OSS. At the time, the rising emphasis on knowledge translation was relatively new. It has since become firmly enshrined across all aspects of health research funding, clinical care guidelines and government policy. While the terms used to describe KT have multiplied and evolved, many of its key features arguably remain the same in the more contemporary practices of EBM. I theorize it then and now as a text that is the managerial arm of EBM.

Health care in Canada, at the time of this study, was in a particular era of emphasis on change and improvement (Health Canada, 2003; Health Council of Canada, 2008). The concurrent sense of urgency around implementing best evidence care could be read in both medical and media accounts calling for greater investment by governments in health care research (Rosenberg, 2003). There was a growing accumulation of scientific and medical evidence and information technologies to help both spread and monitor new evidence, and a focus on developing strategies to urge physicians to implement research findings in their practice. Some critical scholars have argued that inherent in this movement was the

© The Author(s) 2020
F. Webster, *The Social Organization of Best Practice*,
https://doi.org/10.1007/978-3-030-43165-5_1

implicit idea that science can perfect the delivery of medicine through ever more sophisticated drugs and treatments (Traynor, 2002; Walker, 2003).

This focus on change and improvement arose at least in part from the rise of evidence-based medicine. For the past several decades, the field of medicine has been dominated by what has been commonly referred to as the Evidence-based Medicine (EBM) movement. The basic premise of EBM is that by using methods of scientific and epidemiological inquiry, clinicians can deliver best practice medicine. Best practice refers to interventions that are based on results from research that range in hierarchy from meta-analyses of double-blinded randomized controlled trials (RCTs), considered to produce gold standard evidence, to anecdotal or clinical experience. However, as one author has noted, 'The term hierarchy of evidence is a misnomer; the hierarchy is actually a hierarchy of methodologies. That is, it focuses not on the actual results of a particular study or group of studies—in other words, on the evidence they provide for the efficacy of a treatment—but on how that evidence was obtained' (Bluhm, 2005, p. 536). The promise of evidence-based medicine is that it will improve health outcomes for patients. As defined in the literature, the problem arises when individual physicians do not implement best practices in their delivery of care (Cabana et al., 1999; Davis et al., 2003; Graham et al., 2006).

Further, patients and their families are said to have a right to this best evidence treatment (Rosenberg, 2003). To withhold best practice care is considered unethical and uncaring (Davis, 2006; Graham et al., 2006; Grimshaw, Santesso, Cumpston, Mayhew, & McGowan, 2006). Strategies developed with a clear aim to change individual physician behaviour (Armstrong, 2002). Some of these studies focused on physician compliance (Cass, Smith, Unthank, Starling, & Collins, 2003) or adherence (Gifford et al., 1999) and discussed the dilemma of how to change physician behaviour (Lucas et al., 2004). These efforts uncritically accepted that physicians *should* change their practice based on evidence.

Added to this, there was and is pressure on clinicians—physicians, nurses, physiotherapists and other allied health professionals—to also become scientists, to become involved in the production and implementation of new and even better knowledge. The notion that research plays a key role in improving the health of Canadians became increasingly accepted. Rarely were questions asked regarding how patient's participation in clinical research affects their care. As Mykhalovskiy and Weir note, 'Evidence-based medicine creates a demand for clinical trials and thus the recruitment of patients into these trials. What are the effects of the evidence-based market in clinical trials on patients, on physicians and on health care?' (Mykhalovskiy & Weir, 2004, p. 1066).

Although there have been many social science critiques of EBM,[2] and many excellent ones since the time when this study was originally conducted (e.g., Greenhalgh, Howick, & Maskrey, 2014), few studies had empirically studied the social organization of best practice care from a physician standpoint. Through my work, I introduce the Ontario Stroke Strategy[3] as formal medical policy that has been realized in varying institutional and regional settings. What I discovered provides something beyond dichotomous arguments for and against the uses of evidence and beyond abstract theories about how to disseminate evidence to physicians or encourage them to change; instead, I examine what physicians actually do in the everyday worlds of delivering care and making decisions. I began to understand the forms of coordination across different sites that produced variation in care. What emerged consistently from the accounts I gathered is that stroke care was coordinated in ways that often overlooked the everyday conditions under which the individual physician was working. And this coordination masked particular institutional interests that determined the delivery of this acute treatment rather than individual decision-making.

Eccles and Mittman (2006) have described Implementation Science as 'the scientific study of methods to promote the systematic uptake of research findings and other evidence-based practices into routine practice, and, hence, to improve the quality and effectiveness of health services'. Yet this definition overlooks how health care is coordinated in such a way that, despite many clinicians' commitment to prevention and better integration with public health , the majority of funds are directed towards acute care and post-event pharmaceutical therapies. In my work, variation in practice and local context become more than just problems to be solved, but reflected that the narrow band of strategies for which we have evidence does not align with the full range of work that is being provided, or needs to be provided, in hospitals and in the community on an everyday basis. It also begins to identify priorities at the level of hospitals, governments and health charities that are not visible within the stated public claims of 'improving equitable access to care across the continuum'.

Stroke care was the case through which I studied the complex regime that organizes physician's practices in relation to best practice care. Since 1995, the use of a drug known as rt-PA has been defined as best practice for acute stroke treatment. Prior to this, little could be done on an emergency basis to assist the recovery of patients who had suffered an acute stroke. This changed when a drug study produced gold standard evidence that when thrombolytic therapy (rt-PA) was administered to ischemic stroke patients, a benefit could be seen.[4] Experimental results showed that this therapy potentially had the power to halt and even reverse the life-altering neurological damage caused by ischemic stroke. Occasionally it produced an immediate benefit; more usually, this benefit takes place over time. Nevertheless, its potentially transformative effect continues to be likened to the Lazarus Effect by some stroke specialists.[5] There are, however, risks involved in administering it: it carries a 6 per cent fatality rate. In 1999, when rt-PA became established as best practice care for acute stroke in Canada, an infrastructure was created in Ontario to bring it into practice. Promotion of the utilization of rt-PA for acute stroke was accomplished through the development of the Ontario Stroke Strategy, a joint initiative between the Ontario Ministry of Health and Long-Term Care (MoHLTC) and the Heart and Stroke Foundation of Ontario. Through a model that involved creating Regional and District Stroke Centres, best practice care was to be standardized across the province.

A distinctive feature of rt-PA is that eligibility for treatment is determined in relation to the time between possible treatment and the onset of stroke. In addition, only patients with ischemic (rather than haemorrhagic) stroke can be treated, since rt-PA can cause fatal bleeds. A computed tomography (CT) scan must be taken—and professionally read—in order to determine the patient's type of stroke. This involves both technology (the scan itself must be available 24/7) and human resources (radiologist to read the scan). At the time of my study, a core criterion for treatment was stroke onset of less than 3 hours before rt-PA was administered (this time window has been increased to 4.5 hours on the basis of two studies known as ECASS III and the SITS-ISTR registry [Hacke et al., 2008; Wahlgren et al., 2008]). Due to a number of factors, less than 10 per cent of all acute stroke patients are ever eligible for this treatment because of the strict requirements around its use.

In the EBM literature, variations in practice are constituted as a problem to be solved (Rankin & Campbell, 2006). I originally set out to investigate empirically why there was regional variation in physician use of this new evidence-based treatment using the approach of institutional ethnography (IE). IE is an approach to sociology developed by Dorothy Smith. Based on Smith's understanding of the social organization of knowledge,

IE allows for an examination of the complex social relations organizing people's experiences of their everyday lives (Campbell & Gregor, 2002; Smith, 2003, 2005). For Smith, texts mediate and organize people's experiences. In my study, the discourses of both evidence-based medicine and knowledge translation, designed to improve patient care, came into view as managerial tools designed to control the delivery of care. I rendered visible how in fact things worked as they did in real-life settings in a way that linked actual people back to the texts, or discourses, organizing their experiences. In so doing, I was able to uncover some of the assumptions and hidden priorities underlying the current emphasis on translating scientific knowledge in medicine into practice.

I discovered a disjuncture between the best practice treatments developed through clinical trials and the actualities of their translation into practice. In an IE study, disjunctures point to the social relations underpinning the coordination of people's actual work in real-life settings. Here on the one hand was the text-based discourse of EBM and on the other physicians' experiences of the practicalities of conforming to its requirements in the actual situations of their work, often directed through texts which are largely invisible to them. This became the problematic (Campbell & Gregor, 2002) of my study, that is, the general formulation that gave direction to and focused the research and responded to questions such as 'what can we learn from this research? What can it tell us?'

In this study I treat the discourses of both evidence-based medicine and knowledge translation as texts that mediate practice. Understanding—and changing—physician uptake of what is commonly referred to as best practice medicine falls broadly within a field known as knowledge translation. Of course, the terms for this field have proliferated in the past decade, with one study putting the number at 100 (McKibbon et al., 2010) and more recent research, far beyond the time of this study, aimed at what has been called de-implementation (Upvall & Bourgault, 2018). Broadly speaking, KT describes efforts, often undertaken by professional organizations, to increase physician uptake of what are termed best practices. Professional societies develop guidelines and other protocols (Mykhalovskiy, 2003) describing recommended best practices. Knowledge translation is aimed towards understanding how scientific evidence is then translated into clinical practice.

Although the field of KT is inextricably linked to EBM, it has become to some extent discursively disconnected from it. Within the KT field, the focus is always on problems and processes associated with transferring knowledge. In this way, the KT discourse obscures the basis for the knowledge being produced in the first place. The knowledge to be translated, or transferred, is usually developed out of a positivist scientific model. The development of KT techniques, frameworks and strategies presupposes that the knowledge *should* be implemented. The focus is turned away from knowledge production and towards strategies for translating that knowledge into practice. This is an important and unexamined shift as evidence-based knowledge increasingly becomes a 'significant element in the coordination and control of all aspects of work in health care settings' (Campbell, 2010, p. 499). I situate KT as the managerial arm of EBM in order to bring back into view the assumed neutrality of the evidentiary base in knowledge-based medicine.

By focusing on treatment for acute stroke, I explore empirically what actual people are doing in their concrete settings as they produce, promote or try to implement best practices. For Smith (Smith, 1987, 2005, 2006), people's everyday lives can be studied as sites of interface between individuals and a vast network of institutional relations, discourses and work processes. Beginning from the everyday lived experience of those in the field, I am able to trace how best practice for acute stroke is produced by actual people in real settings. I explore how that knowledge is then coordinated across various sites, even when the conditions for uptake are not present in all settings, through the development of the Ontario Stroke Strategy. Finally, I compare the experiences of those delivering care 'on the ground' against the ideal model of care delivery as it has been institutionalized through the textual models developed through the Ontario Stroke Strategy.

The involvement of specific people in developing best practice medicine is rarely obvious. Best practices are developed through a complex set of textual rules that erase the actual people who have been involved in their production. They are often disseminated through texts such as professional guidelines that take for granted and leave unexamined the complex of what is available technologically, the local work conditions, plus the availability and support of other professional staff in carrying out these practices. Within the KT discourse, this complex is subsumed under the heading of context. Context generally refers to any organizational barrier that impedes physician use of best practices. When this local context is recognized, it becomes a problem to be solved (McCormack et al., 2002) insofar as it must be taken into account in designing strategies to change physician behaviour, and for this reason only. At the time of this study, there was very little acknowledgement that these practices might simply not fit the local context, no matter how the settings, or those within them, were manipulated and changed. I set out to ask how this happens. As I began to do so, I discovered that medical specialists in clinical trials taking place in academic hospitals are usually involved in developing best-practice evidence. These trials are largely funded by the pharmaceutical industry, and a portion of the funds received are directed to the university. Due to these aspects of their organization, best practices that are developed are usually acute-care based. Yet the coordination of these complex relationships is largely absent from the EBM discourse.

Technology has also played a large role in how EBM has also evolved over time. Technology is necessary to run massive and multi-site RCTs, which require computerized databases and statistical software. Arguably, outcomes of RCTs have proliferated to such an extent that eventually physicians and nurses could not keep up with the results being produced. While EBM originally began with simple literature searches and review techniques, it now requires systematic reviews, clinical practice guidelines and care pathways. This introduces important extra-local forms of coordination and further obscures how evidence is produced in the first place.

The systematic reviews producing EBM in specific areas rely heavily on statistical probabilities in arriving at their conclusions. Those expected to implement the best practices derived from such studies are acting in relation to particular individual patients and under particular local conditions. The clinician's knowledge may thus come to be seen as being at odds with scientific knowledge (Denny, 1999). My study extends this disjuncture to include the texts that are partially produced by academic medical specialists who participate in clinical trials, and thus are part of producing evidence, and the non-academic physicians who are then expected to implement the practices recommended in those texts. All of these factors change how medicine is practised in local everyday contexts and introduce forms of management which may constrain, or attempt to constrain, professional practice.

Physician practice, of course, cannot be directly controlled by hospital administrators or pharmaceutical companies or policymakers, and for this reason physicians are considered autonomous. Certainly, the EBM and KT literature tends to treat them as a homogenous group. Thus, the notion of the 'physician problem' arises in conversations related to 'how do we get physicians to change their practice?' In January of 2008, I attended a workshop with leading researchers and clinical-researchers to discuss wait times, a by-now recognizable marker of what is 'wrong' in Canadian health care. The speakers at this conference condemned doctors for their alleged inertia. The problem, it was stated by a leading elite physician, was that physicians had too much autonomy. He went on to declare, 'If only General Motors were running this … If we went to GM and saved one million dollars a day, it would be done tomorrow and it would be better for the patient, the doctor and the nurse'. The 'it' to which he refers is best practice medicine. The assumption that EBM practices both save money and are better for both patient and clinician has come to play an important role in the discourse around health care reform. The reference to GM also suggests the valuing of the corporate which is part of the new management of health care. The goals behind knowledge translation efforts are often intertwined with health care reform involving considerations other than the interests of individual patients such as competitiveness, cost efficiency and productivity (Rankin & Campbell, 2006). What, then, is the complex set of social relations underpinning these claims that better health care can be achieved through the development and application of new scientific knowledge? What do these initiatives look like when we explore the lived experience of those providing, and receiving, care? How do the values of competitiveness and cost efficiency factor into those of a positivist and neutral science whose discursive aim is to improve the health of Canadians?

The discourse of the physician problem is troubling, as it directs attention away from the interface between embodied individuals and institutional relations. I am not arguing that physicians don't have power, either collectively through their professional organizations, or in relation to other medical staff such as nurses, within certain medical settings. The assumption behind most strategies designed to address the problem of regional variation is that individual physicians are choosing *on an individual basis* not to incorporate new and 'better' findings in their practice. In contrast, this study draws on the notion of situated practices to describe what happens in the everyday working world of delivering acute stroke treatments across various hospital sites. This term is utilized to draw attention to the everyday work of carrying out what is referred to as best practice in EBM discourse. Through this work, I am able to hook different physician experiences in everyday local work settings to the discourses of evidence-based medicine within those very settings by showing how one group (specialists) contribute actively to what is considered best practice, while another group (community physicians) are expected to implement it. In other words, those who promote best practice are directly involved in developing it in the first place.

This study brings back into sharp view the forms of coordinated work involved in the delivery of acute stroke therapy and reveals the institutional conditions that are taken into account in making a decision whether or not to use rt-PA for the treatment of acute ischemic stroke. My ethnography raises serious questions about some of the concepts embedded within the KT discourse—specifically, the notion of a homogenous universalized physician making decisions autonomously and individually. It also challenges the theoretical basis for KT research, including psychological theories of physician behaviour, and instead shows how conforming to best practices according to the evidence for rt-PA's effectiveness works within the overall organization of health care delivery. I will raise questions about the conflicts of interest that are pervasive within the field of developing knowledge for the evidence base. The ethnography will bring into view actual conditions of providing treatment for ischemic stroke and suggest how the notion of situated practices can be used to investigate the ideal of evidence-based practices.

A disjuncture arises when the best practices derived from evidence developed in the idealized EBM settings are applied to the local setting in which the majority of care is delivered. In order to explicate the social relations organizing the moment at which a decision to use the treatment has to be made, my ethnography begins with the development of the Ontario Stroke Strategy as an idealized model for standardizing acute stroke treatment across the province of Ontario. I then examine the various problems that arise in the implementation of this strategy across various hospital settings, linking these problems back to the discourse and ideology underpinning the physician problem as it arises in relation to the EBM and KT literature.

## NOTES

1. Towards an Integrated Stroke Strategy for Ontario—Report of the Joint Stroke Strategy Working Group June 2000; the Ontario Best Practice Guidelines for Stroke Care; and the results of the Canadian Stroke Strategy Information & Evaluation Consensus Panel, September 2005.
2. For an outstanding history of evidence-based medicine, see Timmerman, S., and Berg, M. (2003). *The gold standard: The challenge of evidence-based medicine and standardization in health care.* Philadelphia: Temple University Press.

3. Over its evolution, the Ontario Stroke Strategy has gone through several name changes, for example, the Ontario Stroke System. For the sake of consistency, I have referred to it as the Ontario Stroke Strategy (OSS) throughout this book.
4. The National Institute of Neurological Disorders and Stroke (NINDS) Study Group reported that 'Despite an increased risk of symptomatic intra-cerebral hemorrhage, treatment with intravenous t-PA within 3 hours of the onset of ischemic stroke improved clinical outcomes at 3 months' (National Institute of Neurological Disorders and Stroke, 1995, pp. 1581–1587).
5. The Lazarus Effect refers to a situation in which a 'full and fast restoration of cerebral blood flow in proximity to the initiation of intravenous tissue plasminogen activator (IV tPA) treatment occurs' (Yarovinsky, Eran, & Telman, 2015, p. 179).

## REFERENCES

Armstrong, D. (2002). Clinical autonomy, individual and collective: The problem of changing doctors' behaviour. *Social Science & Medicine, 55*, 1771–1777.

Bluhm, R. (2005). From hierarchy to network: A richer view of evidence for evidence-based medicine. *Perspectives in Biology and Medicine, 48*, 535–547.

Cabana, M., Rand, C. S., Powe, N. R., Wu, A. W., Wilson, M. H., Abboud, P. C., et al. (1999). Why don't physicians follow clinical practice guidelines? A framework for improvement. *Journal of the American Medical Association, 282*, 1458–1465.

Campbell, M. (2010). Institutional ethnography. In I. Bourgeault, R. Dingwall, & R. De Vries (Eds.), *Sage handbook of qualitative health research*. Los Angeles: Sage.

Campbell, M., & Gregor, F. (2002). *Mapping social relations: A primer in doing institutional ethnography*. Aurora, ON: Garamond.

Cass, H. D., Smith, I., Unthank, C., Starling, C., & Collins, J. E. (2003). Improving compliance with requirements on junior doctors' hours. *British Medical Journal, 327*, 270–273.

Davis, D. (2006). Continuing education, guideline implementation, and the emerging transdisciplinary field of knowledge translation. *Journal of Continuing Education in the Health Professions, 26*, 5–12.

Davis, D., Evans, M., Jadad, A., Perrier, L., Rath, D., Ryan, D., et al. (2003). The case for knowledge translation: Shortening the journey from evidence to effect. *British Medical Journal, 327*, 33–35.

Denny, K. (1999). Evidence-based medicine and medical authority. *Journal of Medical Humanities, 20*, 247–263.

Eccles, M. P., & Mittman, B. S. (2006). Welcome to implementation science. *Implementation Science, 1*(1). https://doi.org/10.1186/1748-5908-1-1

Gifford, D. R., Holloway, R., Frankel, M. R., Albright, C. L., Meyerson, R., Griggs, R. C., et al. (1999). Improving adherence to dementia guidelines through education and opinion leaders. *Annals of Internal Medicine, 131*, 237–246.

Graham, I., Logan, J., Harrison, M. B., Straus, S. E., Tetroe, J., Caswell, W., et al. (2006). Lost in translation: Time for a map? *Journal of Continuing Education in the Health Professions, 26*, 13–24.

Greenhalgh, T., Howick, J., & Maskrey, N. (2014). Evidence based medicine: A movement in crisis? *British Medical Journal, 348*, g3725.

Grimshaw, J. M., Santesso, N., Cumpston, M., Mayhew, A., & McGowan, J. (2006). Knowledge for knowledge translation: The role of the Cochrane Collaboration. *Journal of Continuing Education in the Health Professions, 26*, 55–62.

Hacke, W., Kaste, M., Bluhmki, E., Brozman, M., Dávalos, A., Guidetti, D., et al. for the ECASS Investigators. (2008). Thrombolysis with Alteplase 3 to 4.5 hours after acute ischemic stroke. *New England Journal Medicine, 359*, 1317–1329.

Health Canada. (2003). *First ministers' accord on health care renewal.* Ottawa, ON: Author. Retrieved May 2, 2008, from http://www.hc-sc.gc.ca/hcs-sss/delivery-prestation/fptcollab/2003accord/index-eng.php

Health Council of Canada. (2008). *Rekindling reform: health care renewal in Canada, 2003–2008.* Toronto, ON: Health Council of Canada.

Lucas, B. P., Evans, A. T., Reilly, B. M., Khodakov, Y. V., Perumal, K., Rohr, L. G., et al. (2004). The impact of evidence on physicians' inpatient treatment decisions. *Journal of General Internal Medicine, 19*, 402–409.

McCormack, B., Kitson, A., Harvey, G., Rycroft-Malone, J., Titchen, A., & Seers, K. (2002). Getting evidence into practice: The meaning of context. *Journal of Advanced Nursing, 38*, 94–104.

McKibbon, K. A., Lokker, C., Wilczynski, N. L., Ciliska, D., Dobbins, M., Davis, D. A., et al. (2010). A cross-sectional study of the number and frequency of terms used to refer to knowledge translation in a body of health literature in 2006: A Tower of Babel? *Implementation Science, 5*, 16. https://doi.org/10.1186/1748-5908-5-16

Mykhalovskiy, E. (2003). Evidence-based medicine: Ambivalent reading and the clinical recontextualization of science. *Health: An Interdisciplinary Journal for the Social Study of Health, Illness and Medicine, 7*, 331–352.

Mykhalovskiy, E., & Weir, L. (2004). The problem of evidence-based medicine: Directions for social science. *Social Science & Medicine, 59*, 1059–1069.

National Institute of Neurological Disorders and Stroke rt-PA Stroke Study Group. (1995). Tissue plasminogen activator for acute ischemic stroke. *New England Journal of Medicine, 24*, 1581–1587.

Rankin, J. M., & Campbell, M. L. (2006). *Managing to nurse: Inside Canada's health care reform*. Toronto, ON: University of Toronto Press.

Rosenberg, R. N. (2003). Translating biomedical research to the bedside. *Journal of the American Medical Association, 289*, 1305–1306.

Smith, D. (2003). Making sense of what people do: A sociological perspective. *Journal of Occupational Science, 10*, 64–67.

Smith, D. E. (1987). *The everyday world as problematic: A feminist sociology*. Toronto, ON: University of Toronto Press.

Smith, D. E. (2005). *Institutional ethnography: A sociology for people*. Lanham, MD: AltaMira.

Smith, D. E. (Ed.). (2006). *Institutional ethnography as practice*. Lanham, MD: Rowman & Littlefield.

Traynor, M. (2002). The oil crisis, risk and evidence-based practice. *Nursing Inquiry, 9*, 162–169.

Upvall, M. J., & Bourgault, A. M. (2018, April 25). De-implementation: A concept analysis. *Nursing Forum*. https://doi.org/10.1111/nuf.12256

Wahlgren, N., Ahmed, N., Dávalos, A., Hacke, W., Millán, M., Muir, K., et al. (2008). Thrombolysis with alteplase 3-4.5 h after acute ischemic stroke (SITS-ISTR): An observational study. *Lancet, 372*, 1303–1309.

Walker, K. (2003). Why evidence-based practice now? A polemic. *Nursing Inquiry, 10*, 145–155.

Yarovinsky, N., Eran, A., & Telman, G. (2015). Prompt recanalizaton of basilar artery (Lazarus Effect) in patient with acute ischemic cardioembolic stroke in spite of relatively late start of fibrinolytic therapy. *Journal of Vascular Medicine and Surgery, 3*(1), 1–3. https://doi.org/10.4172/2329-6925.1000179

# CHAPTER 2

# Developing the Ethnographic Study

Like many other institutional ethnographic studies, my own begins with what has been called an 'autobiographical research narrative' (Mykhalovskiy, 1999). In much research, the researcher's presence is treated as a bias that must be overcome (Campbell & Gregor, 2002). As Smith (2006) notes,

> An IE does not rely on notions of objectivity in order to produce 'validity'. However, it does strive to 'produce accurate and faithful representations of how things actually work; it must be truthful. Political commitment here enforces the researcher's responsibility to get it right'. It must remain faithful to the accounts provided by people of their lived experience while going beyond that experience to explicate how that experience happened as it did. (p. 42)

In February 2002 I was hired by a large urban hospital into the role of community planning coordinator for a Regional Stroke Centre in Ontario, Canada. I came to this work as a non-clinician with a Master's degree in sociology whose professional background included health services research and project management as well as administrative and adjunct roles in universities. I was unaccustomed to hospitals, hospital organization and, more specifically, the field of stroke care. For me, the learning curve was significant. I struggled to learn medical and health system terms, such as ischemic, endarterectomy and care pathways, among many others, as I attempted to make sense of this new world I had entered. As a sociologist, this allowed me a perspective on what I was observing

© The Author(s) 2020
F. Webster, *The Social Organization of Best Practice*,
https://doi.org/10.1007/978-3-030-43165-5_2

that was different from the informed experience of those around me. This would change, however, as I slowly become part of the environment in which I worked. Being immersed in the environment which I was studying had implications for the way I conducted and analysed my research (see the section on 'Institutional Capture').

In my role, I was charged with the task of establishing District Stroke Centres (DSCs), funded by the provincial Ministry of Health, in seven communities in Ontario. One of the primary designation criteria for becoming a District Stroke Centre was the ability to deliver acute stroke treatments (see Appendix A). This involved the capacity to administer thrombolytic therapy (rt-PA) for acute strokes. Each centre was also to provide best practice stroke care across the care continuum to a larger region comprising community hospitals, long-term care centres and rehabilitation centres, to name but a few.

The care continuum refers to the various sectors involved in providing care, for example, primary care, acute care, and rehabilitation and community services. I did not originally consider that the continuum of care did not exist beyond textual accounts developed to discursively organize the goals of the strategy, nor did I suspect that there were significant differences in resources between the various settings where care took place. It seemed reasonable to me that the entire strategy could be organized around the delivery of acute care without in any way affecting how that care was equitably delivered. The work of establishing District Stroke Centres (DSCs primarily involved setting up local committees with representation from across the continuum of care. Through the local District Health Councils (DHCs),[1] I identified key players in each community across the continuum—leadership from health promotion through to acute care on through patient community re-integration—and then invited them to meetings to explain the Ontario Stroke Strategy (OSS) and to seek their participation on the committee. These meetings were generally held at the DHCs or in a hospital boardroom. In each community, I presented community profiles that related to the capacity for stroke care and asked stakeholders to identify any information or resource gaps. These profiles were largely based on a survey conducted by the Institute for Clinical Evaluative Sciences (ICES) to determine what type of technology and human resources existed in each community related to stroke care (Tu & Porter, 1999).

Rarely did the data I presented fit the experience of those I sought to represent. At each meeting people expressed that they were not used to working with others from different disciplines; for example, physiotherapists have little experience working with neurologists and family physicians rarely attended meetings. The evaluation forms collected at each meeting consistently revealed that few people felt that the numerically generated data—which identified a community's strengths and weaknesses in relation to stroke care—represented their concerns or experiences. This disjuncture was puzzling to me.

The Regional Stroke Centre into which I was hired originally consisted of a regional stroke coordinator, to whom I reported, and whose job it was to promote best practice and provide care across a large geographic region. A medical director lent his medical expertise and credibility to the region, although he was not involved in the planning work of the region. We were all housed within the Academic Health Sciences Centre in our city, although in separate offices on different floors.[2]

In order to be able, in some way, to serve the needs of its large and complex geographic region, a Regional Steering Committee was established with representation from across the continuum of care and across several counties. This involved over nine counties and eventually also included five District Stroke Centres which were designated in the southwest region. Thus, the geographic area to be covered by one Regional Centre consisting of two full-time staff and one part-time medical director comprised 105 long-term care facilities, 9 Community Care Access Centres and Public Health Units, 3 Base Hospitals, over 40 hospitals and 3 District Health Councils.[3] The model, then, presupposed capacity on the part of the Regional Stroke Centre—located in just one hospital, despite its implied regional responsibilities—to establish and maintain concrete relationships between the region and all the organizations it served.

Within the hospital where I worked, I was also part of a large and highly qualified acute stroke team, which included several international fellows,[4] all of whom were neurologists, and one nurse practitioner. Two other nurses worked full-time on stroke-related clinical studies; I refer to them as 'study nurses' throughout this book. The acute stroke team was distinct from the Regional Stroke Centre staff. Part of the everyday work of the hospital was to attend rounds which were often held over the lunch hour with food supplied by a pharmaceutical company. At these weekly stroke rounds, various expert physicians or residents presented an interesting case or research, or both.

When a patient arrived at the emergency department in our hospital and was identified as having a stroke, a patient stroke protocol was implemented. One of the several stroke specialists, who were fellows, would be paged. A study nurse, whose sole responsibility was to assist in conducting research studies, would be notified to support the physician and also to speak to the family so as to assess the time the patient was 'last seen well' and to obtain consent for both rt-PA and inclusion in a study. At the patient bedside, using a scale that measured the stroke level of severity, the patient would be assessed to determine the severity of his or her stroke. The patient would be quickly transported to the computed tomography (CT) scanner by staff and while she or he was receiving a scan by a technician, the radiologist would be called, as well as one of the neurologists who were considered more senior. After quickly interpreting the scan and identifying the patient as ischemic or haemorrhagic, any patient who was identified as having an ischemic stroke within the 3-hour window would have an IV tube inserted into her or his arm to administer the rt-PA. The patient would then be transported to an organized stroke unit where she or he would receive care from several highly trained and experienced nurses and physicians. I did not realize initially that not all hospitals had acute stroke units.

Both the process and the outcomes seemed miraculous to me. I was quite impressed by the efficiency of the system and also by the science behind the rt-PA drug. Why, I thought, wouldn't every physician want to deliver this potentially miraculous cure to his or her patients? As I became more familiar with my particular acute care setting and with the impact of stroke on people's lives as well as their families and caretakers, this increasingly puzzled me. I attended national and international scientific conferences and learned how drug companies were attempting to find new drugs that would extend the amount of time rt-PA could be administered. Other researchers called for new and better imaging (Silver et al., 2001). The reliance on pharmaceutical and technological advances for treatment struck me as innovative and exciting.

At the same time, I also continued my work across the Southwestern Ontario region, meeting with nurses and physiotherapists and physicians working in community hospitals. As I drove for hours across country roads to visit community hospitals, I became quickly aware of the limited resources and the lack of acute care specialists in smaller hospitals. On my way to one meeting, I stopped for a sign that read 'Horse and Carriage Crossing' and was struck by the physical, visceral differences between smaller community hospitals and the large, urban teaching centre in which I was located. Some of the assumptions hidden within the highly specialized environment in which I worked began to emerge in my consciousness. Smith has introduced the notion of 'bifurcated consciousness' (Smith, 1987) in describing her disparate roles as mother and academic. In a similar manner, I began to experience my physical self out in the rural and semi-rural communities as being in contradiction to my administrative role to help the community hospitals expand their use of rt-PA for acute stroke. In my own unease in subordinating what I was discovering experientially to the institutional discourse of implementing the Ontario Stroke Strategy (OSS) as standardized best practices, I was beginning to touch on those forms of ruling that are mediated by texts (Smith, 2005).

I began to sense, although not yet fully understand, that some relation existed between the ideal world of the evidence-based medicine (EBM) movement which produced the best practice of rt-PA for stroke and the settings in which the textually specified best practices were taken up in situated practice. And so I began my ethnography, in my insider/outsider role as a non-clinical research associate working with a stroke team for three years in Ontario, by speaking with physicians in different settings about how they went about deciding to give, or not give, rt-PA for acute stroke. In so doing, I began to move away from the theories and debates about physician uptake of best practice medicine to explore what they and others were actually doing in their work. My task as an institutional ethnographer was to *find the social*—meaning the forms of organization coordinating people's work—in the accounts being provided to me.

## INSTITUTIONAL ETHNOGRAPHY

Institutional ethnography (IE) was developed by feminist sociologist Dorothy Smith. Smith refers to this approach as a method of inquiry that uses people's everyday experiences as the starting point for an exploration of the often-invisible social relations underpinning or organizing their experiences. It is a highly sophisticated approach based on her understandings of the social organization of knowledge as well as the understandings of other IE practitioners (Campbell & Manicom, 1995). The central premise of IE is that we live in a text-mediated world in which relations of ruling are accomplished through texts that coordinate our activities with those of others, although this is rarely visible to us from our particular standpoints. Understanding the social world requires taking up a specific position as a starting point from which to begin to explore how things are put together the way that they are. In this sense, IE is sampling an institutional *process* rather than a *population* and provides an alternative to the highly abstract and theoretical accounts of the world often provided through mainstream sociology (Smith, 2005).

The standpoint I take up here is that of physicians working in cities and smaller communities and who are involved in delivering rt-PA for acute stroke. The physicians with whom I spoke are held responsible for making clinical decisions in the use of rt-PA for acute stroke. However, while I begin from their perspective, physicians are not the objects of my investigation. Unlike most qualitative methods, these experiences constitute an entry rather than an end point into my exploration of the organization of stroke care. In this way, an IE study cannot be subsumed under the category of qualitative research although it makes use of its methods. Locating an institutional standpoint within the experiences of physicians as a framework of relevance allowed me to direct my gaze to how things were organized in such a way as to standardize a textually established best practice that had to be enacted across multiple locations. Yet these Ontario locations differed widely in the social and organizational conditions under which best practice could be delivered and hence in the empirical practicalities of treating stroke cases using rt-PA.

Standpoint in IE evolved from Harding's use of the term (1988) and refers to the subject positioner of the knower (Smith, 2005). Yet in IE it is distinct from Harding's concept and also from the usage of the term by theorists such as Nancy Hartsock (1998) in that it does not privilege a position within a category of gender, class or race, but instead creates a 'point of entry into discovering the social'. As Smith describes, 'the institutional ethnographer works from the social in people's experience to discover the presence and organization of [ruling relations] in their lives and to explicate or map that organization beyond the local of the everyday' (Smith, 2005, pp. 10–11).

For Smith, texts mediate and organize people's experiences. In my study, the discourses of both evidence-based medicine and knowledge translation (KT), designed to improve patient care, come into view as managerial tools designed to control the delivery of care. I rendered visible how in fact things worked as they did in real-life settings in a way that links back actual people to the texts, or discourse, organizing their experiences. In so doing, I am able to uncover some of the assumptions and hidden priorities underlying the current emphasis on translating scientific knowledge in medicine into practice.

There were several texts that entered into the organization of care in the settings I studied. In addition to the 'Blue Book', there were care pathways and stroke protocols, for example.[5] The Blue Book was written by a working group that included representatives from the Ontario Ministry of Health and Long-Term Care, the Heart and Stroke Foundation Ontario (HSFO) and the Institute of Health Evaluative Sciences, among others, and outlined what the best practice standards should be across the stroke care continuum in Ontario (Joint Stroke Strategy Working Group, 2000). Yet for me, the discourses of EBM and KT were the texts that drove and organized the implementation of these other texts as the 'best practice' that should inform care. Smith has referred to these as 'boss texts' so as to capture their governing character (Griffith & Smith, 2014, p. 11). The institutional ethnographic use of the concept of discourse draws on the work of Michel Foucault (1980). Institutional ethnography has extended Foucault's concept that is restricted to what is written, spoken or thought to actual 'translocal relations coordinating the practices of definite individuals talking, writing, reading, watching, and so forth, in particular local places at particular times' (Smith, 2005, p. 224). People both participate in discourse and reproduce it.

Evidence-based Medicine (EBM) refers to a widely used approach to medical practice that promotes the use of what is known as evidence, produced through particular technologies of both science and epidemiology, in medical decision-making. Knowledge translation (KT) is a discourse that develops strategies and approaches designed to encourage clinicians to make use of this evidence in their practice. Both EBM and KT rely on certain texts, such as care pathways and protocols that are used in health care settings. Rankin and Campbell have argued that these texts of EBM are part of the new public management (NPM) which increasingly relies on 'the expertise of information professionals, auditors, and managers who generate and use a different kind of expertise from that of health professionals' (Rankin & Campbell, 2006, p. 10). NPM 'involves the imposition of managerial regimes modelled on those already operative in the sphere of private enterprise' (Griffith & Smith, 2014, p. 5).

The field of knowledge translation introduces a discourse that extends that of evidence-based medicine at the same time as it obscures its relationship to the latter. Social science critiques of EBM are not being applied to knowledge translation, but rather social science has been taken up in the *promotion* of knowledge translation. In the KT literature, the emphasis and focus is increasingly on *how* to transfer knowledge. The emphasis on getting knowledge into 'action' (Graham et al., 2006) tends to reduce and limit the opportunities for debates about what *type* of knowledge (i.e., experiential, scientific and clinical) has been excluded from the accepted evidentiary knowledge base. It also creates the misleading impression that evidence, as it is defined in the EBM literature, exists for all procedures.

Proponents of KT are sometimes quite explicit in their adoption of language from business models that have informed broader health care reform and in their uncritical belief in research evidence, coupled with a clear intent to change physician behaviour (Armstrong, 2002). For example, some of these studies focus on physician 'compliance' (Cass, Smith, Unthank, Starling, & Collins, 2003) or 'adherence' (Gifford et al., 1999) and 'how to change physician behavior' (Lucas et al., 2004), and even proposed strategies that are active, multiple and aimed at overcoming barriers to change (Davis, 2006). These efforts uncritically accept that individual physicians should change their practice. Some of these attempts have included the development of care pathways, protocols and other standardized texts for treatment. These text-based forms of control have given rise to tensions between the clinical autonomy of physicians and non-physician experts.

These approaches direct attention away from the interface between embodied individuals and institutional relations. Health services research, in which much knowledge translation research is developed, is an evaluation-based knowledge (Mykhalovskiy, 1999). Through the evaluative gaze of health services research, current health care practices not supported by evidence-based medicine are often viewed as 'irrationality and potential waste' (Mykhalovskiy, 1999, p. 2). Under this gaze, the physician problem arises through the KT discourse.

EBM has evolved over time, and a large part of its growth has been fuelled by the availability of technology. Technology is necessary to run massive and multi-site randomized controlled trials (RCTs), which require computerized databases and statistical software. Arguably, outcomes of RCTs have proliferated to such an extent that physicians and nurses could not keep up with the results being produced. While EBM originally began with simple literature searches and review techniques, it now requires systematic reviews, clinical practice guidelines and care pathways.

## The Study

I spoke with physicians in various hospital settings about their decisions regarding whether or not to use rt-PA for acute stroke.[6] This was important in order to begin to understand the activities of physicians doing this work. Best practice is a discourse that translates EBM into a guide for how physicians should proceed. The texts it produces include professional guidelines, protocols and care pathways. But a physician has to make a decision in an actual work situation and be responsive to its realities as he or she enacts them. Most research-based descriptions of physician decision-making are abstract accounts that are not connected to the actual work that they engage in or else refer to individual psychological explanations for physician behaviour (Bonetti et al., 2003; Eccles et al., 2007; Green & Seifert, 2004). The physicians and other health care providers I spoke with described for me their knowledge of their own work and its part in the process of care. People can describe to you what Smith (2005) refers to as 'work knowledge'. It is important to differentiate this from 'perspectives'. Work knowledge is what people are able to tell you about their everyday practices and how they are oriented to the work of others active in the same process.

Institutional ethnography emphasizes people's work and how it is coordinated with that of others. The concept of work refers to what people actually do in particular places, under definite conditions and with definite resources (Smith, 2003, p. 65). This approach eliminates the distinction between paid and unpaid work and includes activities that we do not normally consider part of work. For example, in Tim Diamond's (1992) ethnography of seniors' residences in Chicago, he describes two elderly women sitting looking at the elevator waiting for breakfast to arrive. Waiting, Diamond tells us, is work that patients perform. This concept of work and of work knowledges is what the ethnographer draws on in talking to informants. Among other relevances, it opens the possibility of exploring informal aspects of care that are rarely accounted for in professional practice guidelines and of analysing the role of texts and writing in the work physicians perform. In the case of the physicians who are the focus of this study, it encompasses a range of everyday strategies (e.g., negotiating repatriation of patients and initiating a patient's enrolment in a randomized controlled trial); practices (e.g., reading CT scans with or without the support of radiologists) and activities (e.g., filling out forms and making phone calls). This is an important research focus because when the work of physicians is not fully understood, their engagement in 'best practice', whether by developing evidence or failing to implement it, becomes less visible.

In institutional ethnography, the interviews are not end points in themselves but instead starting points which allow me to begin to analyse the context in which the use of rt-PA for acute stroke actually takes place and to understand the features of institutional work that inform the organization required to deliver this care. As such, interview material is not the raw data to be worked into an account; rather, 'When interviews are used in this approach, they are used not to reveal subjective states, but to locate and trace the points of connection among individuals working in different parts of institutional complexes of activity' (DeVault & McCoy, 2006, p. 18). While the physicians, other health care providers and patients and their families I spoke with represented different standpoints, they did not represent different perspectives, which is a concept that individualizes each experience. The IE method is instead designed to capture, through the standpoint of the participants, the invisible institutional coordination of their work that can be heard through participant's accounts.

The physicians I spoke with worked in settings with different institutional characteristics. Some were from urban, academic teaching centres, host to a Regional Stroke Centre; some were family physicians working in emergency departments in semi-rural areas; and at both District and Regional Stroke Centres. They were also from different professional backgrounds; some were neurologists or stroke fellows; others were internal medicine specialists, and some were family physicians, rehabilitation specialists or physiatrists. For the purposes of anonymity and clarity, I have referred to them as specialists or district/community physicians throughout this book in order to distinguish both the location where they work and their degree of specialization within medicine. The term specialist refers to (or may occasionally be described as) physicians with specialization, usually in neurology, or clinician-scientists who work in Academic Health Sciences Centres (AHSCs) where Ontario's Regional Stroke Centres are housed. The term community physician refers to physicians, generally without specialization, who work in either District Stroke Centres or community hospitals.

Institutional ethnography looks for something outside of the experiences of key informants which is largely invisible to them and yet which enters into and coordinates their work with those of others of whom they may not be aware. Exploring relations beyond the physicians' experience meant learning from others who were in various ways at work in the same settings. Hence, while I started with physicians' descriptions, I also conducted approximately 40 interviews over two years with other health care providers, patients, and their family members across various sites in Ontario.

## THE PROBLEMATIC

The notion of the problematic in institutional ethnography (Rankin, 2004; Smith, 1987, 1999, 2005) does not refer to what those within the setting would necessarily describe as the problem they are facing at any given moment. It is a technical term that Smith and others use to describe that which is troubling beyond the range of what those working within a particular system can see. It provides the link between what is experienced at the local level and the extra-local forms of coordination informing it. Those I interviewed identified the problem as they see it as the variation in the provincial rates of provision of rt-PA, as I also did initially. However, I realized there were other troubling issues. While EBM may generate best practices, these practices have not been readily translated into local practices. Knowledge translation emerged as a field, and as a discourse, that focuses on the translation of EBM into practice. Its emphasis on the process of transferring knowledge directs attention from how that knowledge was produced.

There is also a strong focus on physicians as themselves constituting the problem when knowledge isn't transferred successfully. In much the way that patient compliance has been both advocated and critiqued, there has been increasing discussion of physician compliance in relation to best practice medicine. Physicians in the community setting are often the intended audience of strategies designed to control their practice. The notion of a change agent has been introduced to describe a person whose role is to advocate for system change; this has been a notable aspect of the Ontario Stroke Strategy (Black, Lewis, Monaghan, & Trypuc, 2003; Hakim, 2007; Lemieux-Charles, McGuire, & Blidner, 2002). The change agent's work is largely accomplished through texts such as care pathways and stroke protocols that still target individuals. However, the most widely used strategies to change practice at the time of this study included the following: educational approaches (Billings-Gagliardi et al., 2001; O'Brien et al., 2001, 2007); strategies that utilize opinion leaders and educational outreach (Doumit, Gattellari, Grimshaw, & O'Brien, 2007); the use of guidelines and clinical pathways (Grimshaw, Santesso, Cumpston, Mayhew, & McGowan, 2006); reminder systems and clinical support systems (Wolff, Taylor, & McCabe, 2004); and financial incentives, such as pay-for-performance measures (Mehrotra, Damberg, Sorbero, & Teleki, 2009). A systematic review of these various approaches concluded only that some things seem to work some of the time (Grimshaw et al., 2004).

Physicians who do not deliver what can be identified as best practice are considered a problem by policymakers and administrators, and various educational, psychological or behavioural strategies are developed to encourage them into compliance. Although not a parallel case, Rankin and Campbell (2006) identified how the problems nurses were having with initiating a new work practice were constituted as interpersonal; they were then subjected to such solutions as workshops focused on building interpersonal skills. This diverted attention away from the organizational issues the nurses were experiencing in relation to patient care. In relation to acute stroke, physician work knowledges are trivialized as irrational fear (Katzan, Sila, & Furlan, 2001). I wondered what was being obscured by this particular focus.

IE evolved as a feminist approach to studying the social world and most IE studies have commenced from within the experiences of those with relatively little social power. For many IE researchers, the method provides an opportunity to understand and respond to social oppression at all levels (Campbell & Gregor, 2002) and furthers the goals and values of democracy. For instance, Griffith and Smith studied the experiences of single mothers (Griffith & Smith, 1987, 2005); Pence began her study in the experiences of battered women (Pence, 1997); Mykhalovskiy and McCoy (2002) shed light on the health care work undertaken by patients undergoing therapy for HIV/AIDS.

Physicians are often considered the elite within medicine, especially in relation to other health care workers and certainly in relation to patients. Their standpoint might then seem an unusual position from which to take up an institutional ethnography. This does not mean, however, that there are not issues for physicians in relation to the new forms of ruling that invade earlier, well-defined professional autonomy. These new forms of ruling would include how health care management (in Canada) or health insurance criteria for treatment (in the United States) control physicians' decision-making in various ways; the latter also include those new forms of ruling or governance that have been developed from evidence-based medicine and translated into best practices which increasingly, through such emerging discourses as knowledge translation, put physicians under pressure to conform.

My study brings back into view all the various other people who are involved in the delivery of acute stroke therapy and reveals the invisible institutional factors that influence the use of rt-PA for the treatment of acute ischemic stroke. Stroke is a serious chronic and óften disabling disease that has far-reaching consequences for patients, their families and the health care system. As a non-clinician, I felt humbled by the dedication of those I had the honour to work with for three years within an acute stroke team. I also felt privileged to have been part of the Ontario Stroke Strategy, whose members, from the regional and district managers to the nurse-educators and policymakers, have worked tirelessly to improve the quality of stroke care for those afflicted by this horrible disease. I hope that in some small way my work will be of use to those working within this system of providing care and that the forms of coordination I have been able to render visible will be taken up not as an attack but as an illumination. In the end, what I have tried to do is produce accurate and faithful representations of how things actually work. I have striven to be truthful and hope that in so doing I have lived up to my responsibility to get it right.

## DATA COLLECTION TECHNIQUES

IE shares with other ethnographic approaches similar data collection techniques (Campbell & Gregor, 2002, p. 8). Ethical approval for my study was received from both the local university affiliated with the hospital where I worked and the University of Toronto where I was a student. All interviews were taped and transcribed. Taping interviews is a standard process common to most qualitative studies and is not unique for the IE researcher. As two IE researchers have described, 'Most IE interviewers tape conversations with informants, both as an aid in making notes and to preserve details whose relevance may not be immediately obvious. Taping also usefully preserves intonation and the emphasis that can be heard in people's voices' (DeVault & McCoy, 2006, p. 24). The interviews were transcribed and entered into a software program (MAXQDA).

## THE DATA

IE makes use of several types of data, including interviews, observations and texts. This has been described as first-level data (Campbell & Gregor, 2002, pp. 59–61) and involves careful descriptions and observations of everyday life. Second-level data involves finding the organizational details that are missing from these experiential accounts, for example, relevant policy documents. The physicians with whom I spoke worked in different towns and cities in the province of Ontario. I also conducted approximately 40 interviews over two years with other health care providers and patients and their family members. The health care provider interviews were conducted with nurses, physiotherapists, social workers, nurse-managers, programme managers, Ministry of Health staff and Heart and Stroke Foundation of Ontario (HSFO) officials across various sites in Ontario.

My observations within the field also became data that I used in my study. Because of my particular location within the health care system, I was able to observe and interview everyone involved not only in the delivery of medical care but also in the development of the policies related to the delivery of that care. For example, I was a member of the Stroke Evaluation Advisory Committee (SEAC), the committee evaluating the Ontario Stroke Strategy at the provincial level; had regular contact with officials overseeing the strategy at the Ministry of Health and Long-Term Care; and helped to edit a Memorandum of Agreement (MoAs) between ambulance services and hospital administrations that was developed to allow patients from outside the region to be diverted from the closest hospital to the nearest hospital providing acute stroke services so that they could receive rt-PA. Having contact with others outside of the direct delivery of rt-PA, but involved in its coordination, allowed me to broaden my understanding of the overall context in which the rt-PA debate occurred.

The literature of both evidence-based medicine and knowledge translation and within medical journals is second-level data that is also part of my analysis (Campbell & Gregor, 2002). The idea that social life is discursively organized is a central component of the institutional ethnographic approach (Campbell & Gregor, 2002). In much contemporary scholarship, it is recognized that simply 'going and looking' as a way to conduct ethnography is no longer sufficient. IE allows for the researcher to be attentive to hearing the social organization in people's accounts of their lives. Analysing the discourse of EBM allowed me to then link people's accounts back to that discourse and how it becomes enacted in the social settings of people's everyday lives.

## INSTITUTIONAL CAPTURE

In addition to my interviews, I engaged in participant observation over a three-year period during which time I was part of an acute stroke team. This was, for me, an amazing and fascinating experience. I was truly immersed in my setting and became part of a close-knit group of international stroke fellows and nurses. It also brought its own difficulties in terms of conducting my research. Smith has identified the difficulties inherent in engaging informants in discussion that goes beyond their institutional rationale in which 'the particulars of the informants' local work are displaced by 'the organization's organizational account' (Smith, 2005, p. 156). Smith has developed the concept of 'institutional capture' (DeVault & McCoy, 2006; Smith, 2003, 2005, pp. 155–157) to describe those situations in which both the informant and the researcher are familiar with and speak the same institutional discourse. She notes that the researcher may not be aware of the extent of their immersion in the discourse until she is reading a transcript. In my own situation, while reading a transcript, I remained unaware of an institutional detail embedded in my informant's account until a second reader drew attention to its remarkable detail. In this particular interview with a specialist in an academic setting, he refers to how a patient arrived by helicopter. This reference did not strike me as unusual, as I worked within an academic teaching hospital where this was the normal experience of everyday work. In crossing from the parking lot every day to the hospital entrance, I had to walk directly past the air ambulance landing zone. When a helicopter was landing, we had to stop and wait until it was safe to cross. Very soon this became a normal feature of my everyday experience, and so during this interview conducted early in my study I did not initially mark this feature of the process of care as being notable.

While I sometimes lapsed into institutional language, I also believe that my social location as 'one of the team' facilitated the conversations I had with the physicians, as they did not see me as an outsider and were perhaps less guarded in masking their accounts with professional discourse. The physicians and other clinicians in my study were willing and able to move beyond the professional discourse to describe to me what was actually happening, although this did not often occur until sometime later into the interviews.

Another and important aspect of institutional capture is not just how one is embedded within the discourse, but also, because of the very nature of the approach, how the researcher is positioned in relation to those being studied. In many ways I have felt conflicted writing my critique of the Ontario Stroke Strategy given my deep respect for those I have worked with and for their integrity and accomplishment. I believe that many aspects of stroke care have been improved through implementation of the OSS. The conditions around how and when this happens are not necessarily the same as how they are described in the EBM discourse. In addition, those physicians I have worked with—and continue to work with—are deeply committed to evidence-based medicine as an approach that they believe will deliver the best care that their patients deserve. And in some instances, this is certainly the case.

The same is true for my position with the KT field. Knowledge translation as a field and under whatever label that the practice has been given has become increasingly popular since I first began my study. I have also gone on to become more and differently implicated in its development. Between 2006 and 2008, I was employed by the Canadian Institutes for Health Research (CIHR) as the Assistant Director Knowledge Translation for 2 of the 13 institutes that comprise CIHR. In this unique and interesting role, I was exposed to yet another aspect of the development of knowledge for health care, as I worked collaboratively with others to advance researchers' understanding and use of knowledge translation. Smith has noted that 'insofar as ethnographers are at work in universities or other research bases and are teaching and publishing the results of research, or otherwise making it available to people, institutional ethnographers cannot avoid being part, directly or indirectly, of what we are investigating' (Smith, 2005, p. 206).

Because of this, I have experienced some sense of betraying those with whom I have worked closely in accomplishing specific professional goals. I have been able to draw upon my personal feelings to better understand how EBM and KT are in fact organized discursively as causes for the social good. I am not alone in this experience. The rise of EBM has been likened by some researchers to a religious movement (Denny, 1999; Traynor, 2002). Relatedly, Pope (2003) applies a social movement perspective to analyse the emergence of EBM; using Herbert Blumer's theoretical framework from the 1950s, she describes how the evolution of

EBM meets the criteria he outlines for defining a social movement. Social movements by contesting power highlight power itself, and she views EBM as the site of a power struggle between those within the medical profession, such as between specialists and family physicians, and also between those within the medical profession and those outside, such as Ministry of Health staff or hospital administrators (Pope, 2003). There is tension between basic scientists and clinical scientists, between competing professional organizations (as I will explore empirically later on), between types of physicians and between forms of management based on information systems and experientially and skill-based knowledge. The field of knowledge translation, then, as an extension of the EBM movement, can also be seen clearly as a struggle between those who produce evidence and those who are meant to apply it.

Those caught in these struggles rarely have any sense that they are struggling over sites of contested power. The moral undertones of EBM discourse, as I will elaborate later on, enter into individual conversations in a genuine manner, insofar as people believe in what they are saying. They believe that through the tools of EBM, they will advance patient care. They have no sense that their activities support the interests of, for example, the government or the pharmaceutical industry. The specific nature of IE's focus on what is beyond the visible range of those working within a particular setting, however, allows for an exploration of social relations that does not necessarily challenge the personal integrity of those who support ruling relations through their work.

Understanding this has allowed me to investigate and write up the social in a way that does not divorce it from the embodied lives of those with whom I worked and studied. It also does not limit my attention to them. DeVault and McCoy (2006) note:

> There is no 'one way' to conduct an IE investigation; rather, there is an analytic project that can be realized in diverse ways. IE investigations are rarely planned out fully in advance, identifying research sites, informants, texts to analyze, or even questions to pursue with informants. Instead, the process of inquiry is rather like grabbing a ball of string, finding a thread, and then pulling it out. (p. 20)

My own IE was not well planned out, but rather emerged from the work that I was doing, located within an urban teaching hospital setting and charged with the task of establishing District Stroke Centres in community hospitals. The 'thread' that I was pulling related to my own observations of the primacy of rt-PA in the development of the Ontario Stroke Strategy, as I helped establish District Stroke Centres. I heard, and then increasingly questioned, why this treatment was at the centre of the strategy and why it remained controversial. How, I wondered, did the use of rt-PA for acute stroke come to be accepted as best practice based on medical evidence? What exactly did that mean? What did it presuppose? And why, if it was such a useful therapy, wasn't it more widely used?

This study goes beyond representations of evidence-based medicine to examine the institutional settings, which are presupposed in its findings, and so describes how the relevant settings are actually organized in the realities of Ontario health care. The method adopted does more than disclose disjunctures, where they exist; it also draws attention to the realities of treatment as specific forms of work organization among the various professional specializations involved that has to be done under definite conditions in a definite time period and with variously available technologies.

Eric Mykhalovskiy locates health services research as part of the reform of health care in Ontario in his study of *informed*, a two-page publication developed by the Institute for Clinical Evaluative Studies aimed at an audience of primary care physicians. He notes that physician reading practices become an object of rehabilitation under the new demands of evidence-based medicine. Under this evaluative gaze, physicians are conceptualized as 'indifferent readers' of EBM (Mykhalovskiy, 2003, p. 338). He concludes that critiques of EBM have tended to be abstract. I will in some sense extend Mykhalovskiy's argument to show how different groups of physicians (academic specialists) are involved in the evaluative gaze of other physicians (community physicians). This produces a discourse of the physician problem that constitutes the non-academic physician as the barrier to the provision of best practice care. This notion then directs attention away from how best practices are developed and constructed. It also masks the process by which patients enter into evidence-based medicine, not just as fortunate recipients of best practice care delivered by academic specialists, but also as subjects in clinical trials. I am interested in how the patient's participation in research affects the clinical care that they receive.

This study takes up at the place where the physician not just reads but also develops and then implements EBM into practice. I did not treat the physician as an individual problem to be resolved but rather took up a physician standpoint to begin to explore and understand the forms of coordination informing their work. My study does not enter into the evidence debate as to whether or not the evidence for rt-PA for acute stroke is sound. Nor do I attempt to make claims about individual physician's beliefs, attitudes or psychological characteristics. As such, I do not assume that physicians should or should not implement the best evidence in their practice. Instead, I sought to ask how the everyday happens for physicians the way that it does and to render visible the forms of coordination organizing the work of different people at different places in time and space. I do not make, refute or argue the theory of knowledge translation; instead, I empirically investigate the concrete realities of what people do as they go about their work of delivering acute stroke care. Said another way, the relational aspect of physician application of evidence-based knowledge is the focus of this study. Through my work, I expose the complex set of working relationships, inter-textual relationships and organization of health care that informs physician practice and argue that the increasing focus of KT efforts on changing physician practice obscures the production of knowledge that precedes it.

## NOTES

1. The DHCs have since been dismantled and reconstituted as the Local Health Integration Networks (LHINs). LHINs are now also being reorganized as of 2019.
2. There are several levels of hospitals in Ontario. For this work, I have used the simplified designations of 'Academic Health Sciences Centre' and 'community hospitals'. This distinction refers to hospitals that deliver specialized services and smaller hospitals with fewer resources.
3. The geographic area covered by each Regional Stroke Centre varied depending on its location. For example, there are three Regional Stroke Centres in the Greater Toronto Area, serving a smaller but more populous area. In Northern Ontario, there are two enhanced District Stroke Centres. They are not housed at academic sites, but they offer higher levels of care, such as trauma, so that they can handle the stroke acuity.

4. A fellow is a clinician who has obtained funding to complete additional training, either in clinical care or in research. They are often recruited internationally and tend to be in the early stages of their career.
5. The formal name of this report is 'Toward an Integrated Stroke Strategy for Ontario, June 2000' (Joint Stroke Strategy Working Group, 2000).
6. Pseudonyms are assigned to all participants throughout the book in order to preserve their anonymity.

## REFERENCES

Armstrong, D. (2002). Clinical autonomy, individual and collective: The problem of changing doctors' behaviour. *Social Science & Medicine, 55,* 1771–1777.

Billings-Gagliardi, S., Fontneau, N. M., Wolf, M. K., Barrett, S. V., Hademenos, G., & Mazor, K. M. (2001). Educating the next generation of physicians about stroke: Incorporating stroke prevention into the medical school curriculum. *Stroke, 32,* 2854–2859.

Black, D., Lewis, M., Monaghan, B., & Trypuc, J. (2003). System change in healthcare: The Ontario Stroke Strategy. *Hospital Quarterly, 6,* 44–47.

Bonetti, D., Johnston, M., Pitts, N. B., Deery, C., Ricketts, I., Bahrami, M., et al. (2003). Can psychological models bridge the gap between clinical guidelines and clinicians' behaviour? A randomized controlled trial of an intervention to influence dentists' intentions to implement evidence-based practice. *British Dental Journal, 195,* 403–407.

Campbell, M., & Gregor, F. (2002). *Mapping social relations: A primer in doing institutional ethnography.* Aurora, ON: Garamond.

Campbell, M., & Manicom, A. (Eds.). (1995). *Knowledge, experience, and ruling relations: Studies in the social organization of knowledge.* Toronto, ON; Buffalo; London: University of Toronto Press.

Cass, H. D., Smith, I., Unthank, C., Starling, C., & Collins, J. E. (2003). Improving compliance with requirements on junior doctors' hours. *British Medical Journal, 327,* 270–273.

Davis, D. (2006). Continuing education, guideline implementation, and the emerging transdisciplinary field of knowledge translation. *Journal of Continuing Education in the Health Professions, 26,* 5–12.

Denny, K. (1999). Evidence-based medicine and medical authority. *Journal of Medical Humanities, 20,* 247–263.

DeVault, M. L., & McCoy, L. (2006). Institutional ethnography: Using interviews to investigate ruling relations. In D. E. Smith (Ed.), *Institutional ethnography as practice* (pp. 15–44). Lanham, MD: Rowman & Littlefield.

Diamond, T. (1992). *Making grey gold: Narratives of nursing home care.* Chicago: University of Chicago Press.

Doumit, G., Gattellari, M., Grimshaw, J., & O'Brien, M. A. (2007). Local opinion leaders: Effects on professional practice and health care outcomes. *Cochrane Database of Systematic Reviews* (1). Art. No.: CD000125. https://doi.org/10.1002/14651858.CD000125.pub3.

Eccles, M., Grimshaw, J., Johnston, M., Steen, N., Pitts, N., Thomas, R., et al. (2007). Applying psychological theories to evidence-based clinical practice: Identifying factors predictive of managing upper respiratory tract infections with antibiotics. *Journal of Implementation Science, 2*(26), 1–14. https://doi.org/10.1186/1748-5908-2-26

Foucault, M. (1980). *Power/knowledge: Selected interviews and other writings, 1972–1977.* Ed. C. Gordon. New York: Pantheon.

Gifford, D. R., Holloway, R., Frankel, M. R., Albright, C. L., Meyerson, R., Griggs, R. C., et al. (1999). Improving adherence to dementia guidelines through education and opinion leaders. *Annals of Internal Medicine, 131,* 237–246.

Graham, I., Logan, J., Harrison, M. B., Straus, S. E., Tetroe, J., Caswell, W., et al. (2006). Lost in translation: Time for a map? *Journal of Continuing Education in the Health Professions, 26,* 13–24.

Green, L. A., & Seifert, C. M. (2004). Translation of research into practice: Why we can't just do it. *Journal of the American Board of Family Practice, 18,* 541–545.

Griffith, A. I., & Smith, D. E. (1987). Constructing cultural knowledge: Mothering as discourse. In J. Gaskell & A. McLaren (Eds.), *Women and education: A Canadian perspective* (pp. 87–103). Calgary, AB: Detselig.

Griffith, A. I., & Smith, D. E. (2005). Introduction. In A. I. Griffith & D. E. Smith (Eds.), *Under new public management: Institutional ethnographies of changing front-line work* (pp. 1–21). Toronto, ON: University of Toronto Press.

Griffith, A. I., & Smith, D. E. (2014). Introduction. In A. I. Griffith & D. E. Smith (Eds.), *Under new public management: Institutional ethnographies of changing front-line work* (pp. 3–21). Toronto, ON: University of Toronto Press.

Grimshaw, J. M., Santesso, N., Cumpston, M., Mayhew, A., & McGowan, J. (2006). Knowledge for knowledge translation: The role of the Cochrane Collaboration. *Journal of Continuing Education in the Health Professions, 26,* 55–62.

Grimshaw, J. M., Thomas, R. E., MacLennan, G., Fraser, C., Ramsay, C. R., Vale, L., et al. (2004). Effectiveness and efficiency of guideline dissemination and implementation strategies. *Health Technology Assessment, 8*(6), iii–iv. 1–72.

Hakim, A. (2007). The 2007 Willis lecture: Vascular disease: The tsunami of health care. *Stroke, 38,* 3296–3301.

Harding, S. (1988). *Feminism and methodology* (p. 1987). Bloomington: Indiana University Press.

Hartsock, N. (1998). *The feminist standpoint revisited and other essays.* Boulder, CO: Westview.

Joint Stroke Strategy Working Group. (2000). *Towards an integrated stroke strategy for Ontario.* Toronto: Ministry of Health and Long-Term Care.

Katzan, I. L., Sila, C., & Furlan, A. J. (2001). Community use of intravenous tissue plasminogen activator for acute stroke: Results of the brain matters stroke management survey. *Stroke, 32,* 861–864.

Lemieux-Charles, L., McGuire, W., & Blidner, I. (2002). Building interorganizational knowledge for evidence-based health system change. *Health Care Management Review, 27,* 48–59.

Lucas, B. P., Evans, A. T., Reilly, B. M., Khodakov, Y. V., Perumal, K., Rohr, L. G., et al. (2004). The impact of evidence on physicians' inpatient treatment decisions. *Journal of General Internal Medicine, 19,* 402–409.

Mehrotra, A., Damberg, C. L., Sorbero, M. E., & Teleki, S. S. (2009). Pay for performance in the hospital setting: What is the state of the evidence? *American Journal of Medical Quality, 24,* 19–28.

Mykhalovskiy, E. (1999). *Knowing health care/governing health care: Exploring health services research as social practice.* Unpublished doctoral dissertation, York University, Canada.

Mykhalovskiy, E. (2003). Evidence-based medicine: Ambivalent reading and the clinical recontextualization of science. *Health: An Interdisciplinary Journal for the Social Study of Health, Illness and Medicine, 7,* 331–352.

Mykhalovskiy, E., & McCoy, L. (2002). Troubling ruling discourses of health: Using institutional ethnography in community-based research. *Critical Public Health, 12,* 17–37.

O'Brien, M. A., Freemantle, N., Oxman, A. D., Wolfe, F., Davis, D., & Herrin, J. (2001). Continuing education meetings and workshops: Effects on professional practice and health care outcomes. *Cochrane Database of Systematic Reviews* (1). Art. No.: CD003030. https://doi.org/10.1002/14651858. CD003030.

O'Brien, M. A., Rogers, S., Jamtvedt, G., Oxman, A. D., Odgaard-Jensen, J., Kristoffersen, D. T., et al. (2007). Educational outreach visits: Effects on professional practice and health care outcomes. *Cochrane Database of Systematic Reviews* (4). Art. No.: CD000409. https://doi.org/10.1002/14651858. CD000409.pub2.

Pence, E. (1997). *Safety for battered women in a textually mediated legal system.* Unpublished doctoral dissertation, University of Toronto, Canada.

Pope, C. (2003). Resisting evidence: The study of evidence-based medicine as a contemporary social movement. *Health: An Interdisciplinary Journal for the Social Study of Health, Illness and Medicine, 7,* 267–282.

Rankin, J. M. (2004). *How nurses practice health care reform: An institutional ethnography.* Unpublished doctoral dissertation, University of Victoria, Canada.

Rankin, J. M., & Campbell, M. L. (2006). *Managing to nurse: Inside Canada's health care reform.* Toronto, ON: University of Toronto Press.

Silver, B., Demaerschalk, B., Merino, J. G., Wong, E., Tamayo, A., Devasenapathy, A., et al. (2001). Improved outcomes in stroke thrombolysis with pre-specified imaging criteria. *Canadian Journal of Neurological Sciences, 28,* 113–119.

Smith, D. E. (1987). *The everyday world as problematic: A feminist sociology.* Toronto, ON: University of Toronto Press.

Smith, D. E. (1999). *Writing the social: Critique, theory, and investigations.* Toronto, ON: University of Toronto Press.

Smith, D. E. (2003). Making sense of what people do: A sociological perspective. *Journal of Occupational Science, 10,* 64–67.

Smith, D. E. (2005). *Institutional ethnography: A sociology for people.* Toronto, ON: AltaMira Press.

Smith, D. E. (Ed.). (2006). *Institutional ethnography as practice.* Lanham, MD: Rowman & Littlefield.

Traynor, M. (2002). The oil crisis, risk and evidence-based practice. *Nursing Inquiry, 9,* 162–169.

Tu, J., & Porter, J. (1999). *Stroke care in Ontario: Hospital survey results.* Toronto, ON: Institute for Clinical Evaluative Sciences.

Wolff, A. M., Taylor, S. A., & McCabe, J. F. (2004). Using checklists and reminders in clinical pathways to improve hospital inpatient care. *Medical Journal of Australia, 181,* 428–431.

# CHAPTER 3

# Setting the Stage for Implementing Knowledge: The Ontario Stroke Strategy

Understanding the context in which care is delivered is acknowledged as an important feature of improving the uptake of best practices (Graham et al., 2006). Yet few studies have clearly delineated what the term means or how it influences physician behaviour (McCormack et al., 2002). In combination with context, the term culture is often applied to account for differences between physician groups or between different health care organizations and to study variations in nursing practice (Manley, 2000).

What is actually happening in various settings tends to disappear from view when the abstract concepts of context or culture are applied. For example, Rankin and Campbell (2006) have shown how the idea of a nursing culture obscures real people. An institutional ethnography (IE) analysis starts in the actualities of people's lives as they experience them and from there understand the organization of their work that may be taken for granted (Smith, 2003). I did not want to ascribe differences to the local context but specifically 'preserve people as active and as doing things in definite places and in the time it actually takes' (Smith, 2003, p. 65).

As I have previously outlined, utilization of thrombolytic therapy (rt-PA) for acute stroke in Ontario was promoted through the development of the Ontario Stroke Strategy (OSS), a joint initiative between the Ontario Ministry of Health and Long-Term Care (MoHLTC) and the Heart and Stroke Foundation of Ontario (HSFO). Through a model that proposed the development of Regional and District Stroke Centres, best

© The Author(s) 2020
F. Webster, *The Social Organization of Best Practice*,
https://doi.org/10.1007/978-3-030-43165-5_3

practice care across the care continuum was to be introduced across Ontario. Thus the strategy aimed to be a vehicle for knowledge translation across the province (Lewis, Trypuc, Lindsay, O'Callaghan, & Dishaw, 2006). However, several problems arose in the implementation of this strategy, especially in relation to the model of regional delivery of services. This chapter begins with a brief description of the Ontario Stroke Strategy model, and then it describes how different physicians working in Regional and District Stroke Centres and community hospitals describe both the work that they do in their respective locations and how their work is coordinated with the work of others across the care continuum.

## THE IDEAL OF THE ONTARIO STROKE STRATEGY

In the fall of 1998, the Heart and Stroke Foundation of Ontario launched the Ontario Stroke Strategy (OSS). According to one informant, the Heart and Stroke Foundation had been under some pressure from their supporters to 'do something' about stroke. After piloting three OSS sites, HSFO then evaluated their progress. In order to do this, they provided funding to the Institute for Clinical Evaluative Sciences (ICES) to develop a registry known as the Ontario Stroke Registry.[1] On the basis of this evaluation, commissioned by HSFO, the Ontario Stroke Working Group was formed and the Blue Book report, described in Chap. 2, was produced by a team that included representatives from MoHLTC, HSFO and ICES, among others. The Blue Book outlined what the best practice standards should be across the stroke care continuum in Ontario (Joint Stroke Strategy Working Group, 2000).[2] Following this, a three-year demonstration project was tested and evaluated to pilot a model of regional coordinated stroke care that spanned the continuum of care. The Working Group then made a recommendation to the MoHLTC to provide $30 million a year to what became known as the Ontario Stroke Strategy. The recommendation was approved, and on that basis the Ontario Stroke Strategy was born.

It is worth noting that although evidence-based best practices were integrated into the strategy, there were also pressures from the health care marketplace and the pharmaceutical industry to develop the OSS.

> The pressure to approve and promote rt-PA in Canada was felt by the Heart and Stroke Foundation, a well-recognized organization with a mission of reducing the risk of premature death and disability from heart

disease and stroke by raising funds for research and health promotion. Healthcare providers, especially neurologists and the healthcare market-place, specifically the pharmaceutical industry, encouraged the Foundation to increase awareness of stroke symptoms and the importance of respond-ing quickly with effective treatments. While the Foundation was confi-dent they could increase public awareness, they were concerned about 'the ethical dilemma of increasing the demand for timely and effective care that was not available'. (Black, Lewis, Monaghan, & Trypuc, 2003, p. 44)

A senior official with the Heart and Stroke Foundation whom I inter-viewed told me that the neurologists had first approached them because 'their clinical trials weren't successful because not enough people arrive in time'. There was hope that a government-supported province-wide strat-egy would advance their recruitment of patients for trials.

The goal of the strategy was to provide equitable access to best practice stroke care across the continuum, achieved through the establishment of Regional and District Stroke Centres. The Regional Stroke Centre was designed to support the District Stroke Centres, which in turn was designed to support the smaller community hospitals. The model of care depicted in this figure presupposes a relationship between those working across various sites and across the continuum. In the organizational account described in the Blue Book, the model 'gives community hospi-tals the support they need to establish organized, evidence-based, patient-centred stroke care' (Joint Stroke Strategy Working Group, 2000, p. 94). But what is meant by the support and how is it enacted in everyday work-ing situations?

## DISTRICT STROKE CENTRES

I am sitting in a physician's office in a small semi-rural community. He is telling me about the recent designation of his hospital as a District Stroke Centre. He was an experienced physician who had been practising medi-cine for decades. He discusses with me how health planners and the hos-pital administration feel that they have met the criteria to be a District Stroke Centre without input from physicians. He comments:

I think administration is going one direction, but the department of medi-cine is saying hold on, let's solve the manpower issues here before informing

> the community, as has been done in the newspapers, that you have a stroke centre. We don't have a stroke centre … [The] problem with rt-PA in our community is that the Department of Internal Medicine can no longer provider 24/7 call. We've been defaulting regularly. Quite a few nights every month no internist is on call, so to call this a District Stroke Centre when there is no expertise around to manage stroke is a thing that is really troubling me right now.

In this account, the physician expresses that the community has been informed of the designation of a stroke centre for his institution that he thinks does not exist in practice. District Stroke Centres were designated through a complex process involving the District Health Councils and the Ontario Ministry of Health and Long-Term Care. The decision to so designate a hospital was based on data that indicated the availability of computed tomography (CT) scanners, for instance, or radiologists. According to one administrator I spoke with, nobody within the OSS or at the hospitals would know which institutions would be designated until there was an announcement. As Rankin and Campbell observe, 'accountability in health care is a textual product distinct from what actually happens' (2006, p. 21). In this instance, what counts has led to the creation of a stroke centre that exists only in documents. As the physician points out, 'obviously this will be a TIA clinic [i.e., transient ischemic attack clinic] on paper only; it won't be seeing patients'.

Proponents of rt-PA call upon the evidence-based medicine (EBM) construction of what I have termed the physician problem to explain why some physicians do not make better use of rt-PA for acute stroke; the problem becomes one of non-compliant or unmotivated individual physicians (Eccles, Grimshaw, Walker, Johnston, & Pitts, 2005; Schwartz & Shulkin, 1995). As one leading stroke specialist declared, 'We need to put knowledge into practice. New knowledge is important but the reality on the ground is that patients are not getting the care we know we could provide' (Canadian Stroke Network, 2004, p. 1). The problem, as constructed here, is straightforward: we have the knowledge and just need to put it into practice. There is no awareness of the kind of situation that this physician is describing in which resources are lacking. According to this physician, the failure of a patient to receive organized stroke care in his hospital had nothing to do with his appraisal of the scientific evidence or individual decision-making. As he states it, 'we simply do not have the resources'. He further comments: 'So we're not sure that our outcomes are the same as the administrative outcomes, and frankly I suspect administrative outcomes basically are driven by the dollar'. Outcomes in health care usually refer to the results from research or patient outcomes from treatment interventions. The most frequently used outcomes are morbidity and mortality for determining the efficacy of a particular treatment. This physician is commenting that the hospital administration's notion of 'outcomes' refers to financial outcomes.

He then provides a powerful example of the difference between knowing 'the evidence' and being able to provide the best care. In the following account, he describes various drugs that can be used to help prevent stroke. The best class of drug—Warfarin—requires follow-up to monitor levels in the patient's blood every week. This physician is working in a rural area. Many of his patients do not have a family physician to do a follow-up and that level of care is not provided by the specialist.

> For instance, if I see someone in atrial fibrillation, they should be on or many of them should be on Warfarin to prevent stroke. If there's no one to follow up, I'll compromise that situation and put them on Aspirin because I don't have the follow-up. If you're looking for one of the reasons why we might have difficulties, well, there's an example there of a compromise in patient care, and, no, Aspirin is not as good a drug as Warfarin for stroke; it has some effect, but it's not as good. But because we cannot manage someone on Warfarin safely, then they won't get it.

He knows the evidence—that aspirin is not as good a drug as Warfarin for stroke—but his inability to ensure the patient's proper management means that he prescribes a less effective drug. The physician, then, cannot make his or her decisions exclusively on the basis of what is considered best practice in EBM terms; decisions are made within the context of both local working conditions and of the work of invisible others—in this case, the availability of a family physician to provide follow-up care.

Other staff at the District Stroke Centre believe that problems in setting up a stroke clinic arise out of conflicts between physicians. Jennifer is a young nurse working in the intensive care unit of the same hospital as the physician I interviewed. Her job has recently changed from providing patient care to 'teaching the staff things related to stroke care, best practice care'. In this account, her reliance on the professional discourse related to best practice care is striking. Jennifer tells me that 'if you ask one of the nurses what the Stroke Strategy is, or what it does, they wouldn't have a clue'. Jennifer knows the person who has recently been hired as the district stroke coordinator and through this relationship knows about the OSS. She is not involved with administering rt-PA for acute stroke. However, she has been active in attempts to establish an acute stroke unit and describes for me the problems with establishing it that arise from the different interests of 'our internists and our family doctors'. Jennifer recounts her impressions from a recent meeting regarding setting up a clinic:

> The problem of initially starting the clinic was the internists didn't want it to seem that they were taking another thing away from them [the family doctors]. The family doctors have their backs up that the internists are taking this away from them or that away from them, and when we were planning the clinic, to me, the whole time I was like, it doesn't really matter what's good for the patients, you are just thinking of yourselves and I was really frustrated with the whole process. I thought, we are presenting what's best practice, what has been proven, and you guys aren't doing it, it says right here, best practices … I think they're all very territorial and most of them are older.

But as we talk, Jennifer describes other issues between family doctors and internists. Through the hospital, internists can obtain community care for patients through the Community Care Access Centre. A family doctor, Jennifer tells me, is angry because he has to wait months for his patients to see a dietician, an example of patient benefit taking a lower priority to institutional priorities. Jennifer ascribes his response to this as personal and individual, saying, 'like he had his back totally up about the fact that we were able to accomplish things that he couldn't do through his family practice'. She adds, 'I think these [older] physicians here in this hospital need to be told that they are employees of this hospital and that this is what is going to happen. I guess [it's because] they're mostly older physicians too'. Because of recent changes in training for both physicians and nurses, it is commonly believed that generational differences account for their willingness (or lack thereof) to use evidence-based practices. This issue came up in several conversations I had, with people attributing problems to someone being either young or old. This tendency has been noticed in other studies in relation to other health care professions (Rankin

& Campbell, 2006) and also has not held up to empirical investigation (Schwartz & Hupert, 2003). Jennifer's comments draw attention to some of the divisions between specialists and family physicians.

According to those I interviewed, the OSS was acute based, meaning that most of its focus was on delivering rt-PA, a treatment given at the acute stage in hospital settings. This was driven in part by neurologists in Ontario who needed more patients to participate in the trials for rt-PA. As one administrator said, 'the main focus in the fiscal year of 2002–2003 was to really understand the acute piece, because that was predominantly the major goal. Now we understand the acute care piece, which is well over 65 per cent of the funding. And now we're trying to figure out what to do with the other piece, which is the entire continuum'. This acute care focus may not necessarily reflect the interests of the physicians working in community hospitals who were not involved in these conversations. For many of their patients, the three-hour window for consultation is simply not feasible given the large geographic distances they must navigate and difficulties posed by seasonal weather. Yet when physicians, such as the one quoted above, do not use best evidence medicine, it is sometimes attributed to such factors as the physicians' age, much the way that Jennifer describes her view of the family physicians who were upset that they could not arrange quick access to community services for their patients.

Stroke victims in large urban centres who are treated in teaching or tertiary hospitals are most likely to undergo CT scanning, to be managed according to a stroke protocol based on the latest scientific evidence and to be considered for rt-PA. According to the 2000 report of the Joint Stroke Strategy Working Group, stroke victims in rural or remote parts of the province are less likely to receive this type of care. Given these systemic factors affecting the delivery of care, it becomes clear that providing equitable access to such care rests on more than individual decision-making by physicians. How can community physicians provide best practice care that involves technology and providers, such as radiologists, who simply don't exist? And in what sense, then, is this best practice if it cannot be implemented?

The clinicians I spoke with felt that the OSS was an rt-PA-driven strategy rather than reflecting improved care across the continuum. That is to say, most of its resources are focused on what happens at the acute care stage, that is, rt-PA for acute stroke. One nursing manager told me, 'If you look in here [i.e., in the Blue Book], it's the first printing of that model that you keep seeing. It especially needs to be updated because it's—it's a very hospital acute-based programme initially, there's no question and it was criticized for that, but there's no question that rt-PA lead to all of this for everything and so you know, what the heck'.

Many others echoed the sentiment that although the OSS was acute care driven, it had drawn attention and funding to stroke and improved services in other areas of the continuum. One community physician described the strategy as opportunist:

> My initial impressions were it was driven by rt-PA and that had provided a window of opportunity because it was sexy and it finally gave a tool ... to actually treat stroke. And as time went by it became clearer to the people there that they would need to incorporate other elements as well, prevention, rehab, integration, but my impression of it was, initially, was that it was a[n] rt-PA-driven process and that the rest of it was there to kind of fill in, and I think it was somewhat opportunistic, and we didn't see it as a bad thing.

Others felt that it had done very little to improve care of stroke beyond the acute phase as in the following account of a rehabilitation physician:

> There are management problems, you've got some that are disabled, that need rehab, there's no rehab beds up in the nursing home, they can't speak, you know, there's nothing sexy about it. And it's not anything that anyone can fix.

Another community physician echoes the idea that the OSS continues to be driven by acute therapy and that this focus does *not* add benefit to other areas of care—but instead detracts from them: 'And it's really rt-PA driven, very acute care driven, and there is very little in the way of rehabilitation; I mean, it's kind of a shame'.

## Problems in the Continuum of Care

In addition to the physician I interviewed at the District Stroke Centre that he felt existed 'only on paper', many I interviewed felt that the concept of setting up centres to deliver stroke care was not based on local realities. A nurse-educator working in a community centre who had been hired to work within a District Stroke Centre described finding out that the floor did not even know what the OSS was:

Well, starting was very difficult in that I think we had the understanding that everything was kind of in place and that the hospital had bought into the idea of the stroke strategy [only] to find out that the floor wasn't even really aware that they would start to see stroke patients, nor were the staff prepared for that, and then that there was no infrastructure in terms of having additional allied health [personnel] that were trained in stroke, so basically, you know, we were plunked in the middle of this brand new programme, very excited, and then to find out that really everything was starting from get-go and there was no infrastructure in place for us.

As far as her work was concerned, delivering stroke care was problematic as some of the best practices for stroke also applied to other conditions. She finds it difficult to dedicate herself exclusively to patients who have suffered a stroke when other patients could also benefit from her knowledge and expertise. As she puts it,

Our stroke programme falls under Critical Care, so there's already an educator assigned to the Critical Care programme. So I also work with her, but I'm only supposed to be doing stroke, and it's really hard if you're in a room within a neurosciences programme, and you're trying to do something for your stroke patient and Mr Smith across the way also has paralysis—and yet you're not supposed to really be in there doing stuff that's not stroke specific. But at the same time, you're trying to help the nurses. The information I give about stroke is also very applicable to your head patients who have paralysis. You would use a sling for all your strokes, and I'm doing education or in services on stroke-specific information, but that can be carried over to Mr Smith who had a head injury. So it's really trying to stay very focused on stroke, but at the same time making the information applicable to all the patients on the floor, without necessarily being in all the rooms, seeing all the patients.

In this account, the nurse's work is related to the work of others in the hospital, in this case with the critical care programme educator. The models proposed by the Ontario Stroke Strategy did not take this reality into account in relation to the hiring of nursing educators to deliver stroke education in hospitals. Here we encounter the notion of disease silos, which refers to the recognition that most diseases are treated separately, by different professionals, even though most risk factors are common across most major diseases. In the past decades, in the field of prevention, there has been a movement to speak about chronic care models. Chronic care models are meant to challenge the professional and disease silos that permeate much of medicine.

Several strong organizational factors impede this happening. For example, health charities choose to increase their donation base by focusing on a disease brand. For example, the Diabetes Association raises money by focusing on diabetes; the Cancer Society raises money by focusing on cancer. Similarly, various professional organizations organize on the basis of a particular profession. For example, there is a Canadian Cardiovascular Society; there is a Congress of Neurological Sciences and a Canadian Association of Emergency Physicians. Thus, the various types of physician specialities are not actually formally connected to one another. They read different journals and participate in different conferences.

The physicians who worked outside of the acute care sector felt strongly that the relationship between physicians working with different sectors of the continuum was non-existent. In this sense, the continuity and relationship suggested by the term continuum were misleading. As a primary care physician working at a long-term care hospital said:

> Long-term care is not a popular area of medicine to be involved in. It is not where the fun is, okay. But they have to be cared for, and so some of us who do long-term care actually enjoy what we do, but it's not the ivory tower, it isn't that. You still get to prevent things, do a lot of good medicine. The gap between long-term care and acute hospitals is the Grand Canyon. There's never been good camaraderie between the groups, even among the physicians. And they don't train the students to phone the physician at the nursing home. It's as if it was a long-distance call to Timbuktu.

A community physician specializing in rehabilitation echoed a similar sentiment, saying "all the [money] went to rt-PA, and rt-PA you know is just where the big money is at, in stroke care. It's the sexy thing, but you can only treat a certain percentage of people, and even then the impact is not that great. Whereas rehab has a huge impact, and it is starving".

Relationships across the continuum do not only refer to those between physicians in the delivery of acute stroke therapies. Problems also arise between various professionals, for example, between physicians and nurses or physiotherapists. This becomes evident in the following account. Judy was a physiotherapist working in a small community hospital. In fact, the hospital itself was so small that I drove past it twice before recognizing it as such. Judy provided an account of a situation with acute stroke where she felt the physician was not properly following the guidelines in terms of providing rehabilitation for a patient after experiencing a stroke. The patient was discharged home, which Judy felt was inappropriate. I asked her how she communicated with the physician, and she told me, 'After I assessed [the patient] the first day I documented all that on the chart. I wrote on my notes and I wrote a note on the doctor's board. And I did talk to the patient and his wife and unfortunately there wasn't a bed available then'. Judy comments on why this patient was sent home: 'I think some of it is political … one physician said to me, "Well, it's just so much paperwork"'. In other words, Judy feels that the physician did not want to transfer the patient to rehabilitation because it is an administrative burden. Yet she does not seem to have a relationship with the physician in which she can verbally communicate her concerns. Instead, she must communicate by writing on the doctor's board. This is an example of the lack of relationship not only between physicians but also between physicians and other care providers.

I often found it difficult to identify formal or informal relationships between physicians through my interviews. Most of the physicians I spoke with provided speculations about other physicians. As discussed earlier, this can take the form of physician's general attribution of fear to emergency room physicians as a group, a group that is reluctant to provide rt-PA for acute stroke. For example, a physician working in a District Stroke Centre told me, 'You don't have enough neurologists to deal with primary prevention. The GPs and internists out there don't do it [because] basically they don't have the time'. One specialist made a similar generalization when he observed: 'Poor GPs, they have to know the guidelines on so many things, it's a wonder they keep one or two straight'. A family physician who worked in the emergency department of a community hospital said:

> We're in the front line and we see all this stuff, you know. And I know Dr Big shot and what he does, yea, I've been to a lot of his lectures. And you know, [this] guy's got—I wouldn't say tunnel vision, but they're very focused on what they do. But I'm out here seeing the real people, the first line you know, and that's what I see.

The OSS did recognize that there were problems in the model it proposed of Regional and District Stroke Centres in terms of providing care to smaller community hospitals. They introduced tele-stroke to provide a link between community physicians and physicians working in districts or urban centres. One physician working in the District comments on the extra work this creates. He says:

> A major issue [now] is how a hospital is trying to become a partner with local hospitals, inside and outside the county. And for the first time in 25 years we suddenly get calls from the docs at these hospitals, 'Well you're the internist, I've got this case that someone has shortness of breath or chest pain or maybe a stroke and I want to send them to you'. I don't need that.

For this physician, this new relationship is imposed; it does not arise naturally out of his everyday working experiences of referral. The lack of relationships between various physicians indicates a flaw in how they are conceptualized as a homogenous group.

## Betty's Story[3]

David Sackett, considered one of the leading founders of EBM, defined it as good clinical management supported by the best available evidence, a method that also took into account patient preferences (Sackett, Richardson, Rosenberg, & Haynes, 1997). Despite this wider definition of what constitutes evidence, critical scholars have argued that a more narrow application has been applied that assigns primacy to the randomized controlled trial (RCT) in establishing best practice due to the hierarchy of evidence upon which its application depends (Klein, 1996; Mykhalovskiy & Weir, 2004). Genuis and Genuis (2006) postulate that EBM's emphasis on a hierarchy of evidence has led to what they term a 'reductionist approach' (p. 53). They argue that 'this formal ordering of evidential reliability declares the greater credibility of conclusions drawn from RCT-generated evidence than from conclusions arising from other forms of evidence and that this focus on this hierarchy has promoted a sometimes exclusive emphasis on RCTs' (p. 53). One of the self-described founders of evidence-based medicine, however, reflecting some years later on the assumption that this method would lead to better patient care, admits that 'so far, no convincing direct evidence exists that shows that this assumption is correct' (Haynes, 2002, p. 2).

The lack of relationships between physicians across the continuum has important consequences for patient care. The following account tells the story of Betty, a 60-year-old patient who had a stroke while waiting for a diagnostic test (angiogram). Her experience is an example of the failure of the referral system and of the coordination of care across the continuum. She was the first stroke patient I met in an interview setting, and I found our conversation very moving. We met in her apartment a few months after she had returned home after an extended hospital stay for acute stroke. The lingering effects of her stroke were still visible. Although she lived alone, Betty now had help to assist her with the daily tasks of life—tasks that most 60-year-old women can do without assistance.

Betty had already been identified as a high stroke-risk patient when she suffered her stroke. As mentioned, her stroke occurred while she was waiting for an angiogram, a diagnostic procedure that would potentially have averted her stroke. She had been through several previous transient ischemic attacks, known as TIAs, which often precede a full stroke. Along the way, she had encountered several different types of physicians.

Betty's first contact was with an optometrist. Betty, like many other patients, had problems with her eyesight, but 'didn't connect [her problem] with a stroke'. So she makes an appointment with her optometrist who tells her, 'There is nothing wrong with your eyesight, but I think that you are probably having a TIA'. Betty then decided to visit her family doctor, who put her on an aspirin a day, telling her it would take months to see a neurologist. And he doesn't refer her. Betty describes this:

> So, he just left me on the aspirin a day. Oh, and then I had another problem with the eye. So then I called the cardiologist, and his secretary called me back and she said he said for you to get in to see a neurologist as soon as possible. She said there is a TIA clinic. And I said, 'Oh I didn't know'. So she gave me a phone number and I did call them, and they were saying how long it might take to get in. But, anyway, I called the TIA clinic and then I had somebody from [the specialist's office] call me and give me an appointment—that must have been his secretary. And I saw [the specialist] and the Stroke Team and they said definitely I needed an angiogram. I had really bad signs of having a stroke if I didn't get it done.

However, it was another two weeks before Betty is able to come in for her angiogram. As she tells me, 'I actually had the stroke a few days before my angiogram was booked'. Once again, however, Betty did not recognize the symptoms of stroke. A passer-by sees Betty in distress and calls the ambulance. By the time they arrived, she was feeling much better. They checked her blood pressure and suggested she should go in for a check-up at the hospital. She refused, explaining to me, 'I didn't connect it yet. At that point I wasn't thinking stroke'.

Betty went home and her friend came over. She begins to feel weaker. Her friend contacted the hospital, who instructed Betty to come in to emergency. Betty phoned her son and his wife. Betty recalled that her son and his wife came over. She tells me that 'They were all worried because I didn't look right and I didn't sound right on the phone. My speech had started to slur a little bit'. Betty, however, was unaware of these symptoms; yet at the hospital, she was not diagnosed with stroke. In her words:

> But, at the hospital—it ended up that I came home. They didn't think that I had … They had no beds, for starts, and they didn't think that I was having a stroke at that particular point.

Betty's sense was that the fact they didn't have a bed was connected to her misdiagnosis. This may or may not be true, but it is an interesting observation. She does, however, wish she had been able to stay overnight. She continues:

> I know they had no beds, but they usually keep somebody until they do have a bed. But anyways, the next day, I still had more signs of—I was just generally so tired and couldn't seem to wake up. So my son took me back to the hospital and they put me in a bed, that day, on the Sunday. I was admitted.

In Betty's account, we can see how the lack of clear or formal relationship between various types of physicians seriously impeded her ability to get the timely care she needed. What also emerges from her account is how much work she has taken on in the coordination of her own care. McCoy (2005) and Mykhalovskiy (2008) have referred to this as 'health work' in their study of patients with HIV undertaking anti-viral therapy. Although beyond the scope of my study at the time, the concept of patient-centred care would come to be an ideal which as of 2020 is still to be realized.

## NOTES

1. A key informant tells me that through this registry, the Heart and Stroke has provided $2.5 million to the Canadian Stroke Network (CSN). Ontario receives $1.5 million of that amount. Its remaining money comes from

Industry Canada as part of a programme called the Network of Centres of Excellence. In this way, ICES became part of the institutional relations behind the developing Ontario Stroke Strategy.

2. The formal name of this report is 'Toward an Integrated Stroke Strategy for Ontario, June 2000'.
3. Pseudonyms have been used throughout this book to protect the anonymity of all participants.

## REFERENCES

Black, D., Lewis, M., Monaghan, B., & Trypuc, J. (2003). System change in healthcare: The Ontario Stroke Strategy. *Hospital Quarterly, 6*, 44–47.

Canadian Stroke Network. (2004). *Canadian Stroke Network Newsletter, 4,* 2, 1–3.

Eccles, M., Grimshaw, J., Walker, A., Johnston, M., & Pitts, N. (2005). Changing the behaviour of healthcare professionals: The use of theory in promoting the uptake of research findings. *Journal of Clinical Epidemiology, 58*, 107–112.

Genuis, S. K., & Genuis, S. J. (2006). Exploring the continuum: Medical information to effective clinical practice. Paper 1: The translation of knowledge into clinical practice. *Journal of Evaluation in Clinical Practice, 12*, 49–62.

Graham, I., Logan, J., Harrison, M. B., Straus, S. E., Tetroe, J., Caswell, W., et al. (2006). Lost in translation: Time for a map? *Journal of Continuing Education in the Health Professions, 26*, 13–24.

Haynes, R. B. (2002). What kind of evidence is it that evidence-based medicine advocates want health care providers and consumers to pay attention to? *BMC Health Services Research, 2*, 3.

Joint Stroke Strategy Working Group. (2000). *Towards an integrated stroke strategy for Ontario.* Toronto, ON: Ministry of Health and Long-term Care.

Klein, R. (1996). The NHS and the new scientism: Solution or delusion? *QJM: Monthly Journal of the Association of Physicians, 89*, 85–87.

Lewis, M., Trypuc, J., Lindsay, P., O'Callaghan, C., & Dishaw, A. (2006). Has Ontario's stroke strategy really made a difference? *Healthcare Quarterly, 9*(4), 50–59.

Manley, K. (2000). Organizational culture and consultant nurse outcomes: Part 1: Organizational culture. *Nursing Standard, 14*, 34–38.

McCormack, B., Kitson, A., Harvey, G., Rycroft-Malone, J., Titchen, A., & Seers, K. (2002). Getting evidence into practice: The meaning of context. *Journal of Advanced Nursing, 38*, 94–104.

McCoy, L. (2005). HIV-positive patients and the doctor–patient relationship: Perspectives from the margins. *Qualitative Health Research, 15*(6), 791–806. https://doi.org/10.1177/1049732305276752

Mykhalovskiy, E. (2008). Beyond decision making: Class, community organizations, and the healthwork of people living with HIV/AIDS: Contributions from ethnographic research. *Medical Anthropology, 27*, 136–163.

Mykhalovskiy, E., & Weir, L. (2004). The problem of evidence-based medicine: Directions for social science. *Social Science & Medicine, 59*, 1059–1069.

Rankin, J. M., & Campbell, M. L. (2006). *Managing to nurse: Inside Canada's health care reform.* Toronto, ON: University of Toronto Press.

Sackett, D. L., Richardson, W. S., Rosenberg, W., & Haynes, R. B. (1997). *Evidence-based medicine: How to practice and teach EBM.* New York: Churchill Livingstone.

Schwartz, A., & Hupert, J. (2003). Medical students' application of published evidence: Randomized trial. *British Medical Journal, 326*, 536–538.

Schwartz, S., & Shulkin, D. (1995). Teaching an old dog new tricks. *Journal of General Internal Medicine, 10*, 353–354.

Smith, D. E. (2003). Making sense of what people do: A sociological perspective. *Journal of Occupational Science, 10*, 64–67.

# CHAPTER 4

# The Everyday Practices of Randomized Controlled Trials

It became clear to me through the course of my ethnographic investigation that physicians and nurses are involved in randomized controlled trials (RCTs) as a feature of their everyday work. Anthropologist Helen Lambert noted that evidence-based medicine (EBM) is largely focused on 'the problem of introducing, disseminating, and implementing evidence [i.e., research findings] in clinical practice' (Lambert, 2005, p. 3). That is to say, far less focus has been put upon how evidence is produced and by whom.

In this chapter, I describe what I observed or was told by nurses and physicians about their everyday practices of participating in clinical trials as they go about their work of providing care in academic teaching hospitals. Through these accounts, the invisible social relations underpinning how research and care are coordinated emerge. It becomes increasingly clear that only one group of physicians is in fact part of the development of this knowledge and that this group tends to then promote that knowledge.

## The Clinical Trial in Situated Practice

There is a paucity of empirical description within the knowledge translation (KT) literature regarding how evidence is concretely developed in local situations. As I was looking over my transcripts and field notes, I began to notice that evidence is, of course, produced through various types of research. But the participation of doctors and nurses in the clinical

© The Author(s) 2020
F. Webster, *The Social Organization of Best Practice*,
https://doi.org/10.1007/978-3-030-43165-5_4

arm of that research is taken for granted and unexplored. Research has become part of the norm of the physician and nurse's actual work that is performed on a daily basis in hospitals. The line between clinical care and the work of producing knowledge is often blurred.

The idea that medical evidence is partly developed through clinical trials was one with which I was very familiar and did not particularly examine. I wasn't sure where clinical trials took place but assumed it was 'somewhere out there'; the term held for me some great authority. Yet this changed when I observed the assessment of a patient in an emergency room for thrombolytic therapy (rt-PA). Chapter 5 records the first time I became aware of how integrated research was with the process of delivering care in an academic health care setting. I observed the central role of the study nurse not only in recruiting patients for trials but also in providing highly expert care. At first I took it for granted, as did everyone around me, that the study nurse's purpose in attending this patient is to support the work of the physician, helping to assess the patient's status, finding out critical information from observers as to the timing of the patient's stroke and so on. Although she performs these functions, her purpose in carrying out these activities is to determine whether or not the patient is eligible for participation in an RCT regarding neuro-protectants and to seek consent from the family or patient. In this way, the nurse's work for the study trial means that the patient will benefit from her assistance in the treatment, as these two activities overlap. In a community setting, there are less likely to be study nurses to assist in the work of delivering rt-PA, although there will be other nurses available—but they will not be specifically trained in stroke care. If the patient does not fit the criteria of a particular study, then she or he will not benefit from the presence of this highly trained health care professional. The ethics of this are rarely discussed in the KT or EBM literature.

Conducting clinical research in a hospital setting also impacts the daily work of other health care providers. In one interview, a floor nurse who worked at a Regional Stroke Centre complained to me that one physician's study was conflicting with the operation of the stroke unit where patients were receiving care. As noted, the reorganization of stroke care relies heavily on bypass agreements that allow patients to bypass their home or closest hospital to be taken to a stroke centre offering rt-PA services. This coordination of services is managed through memorandums of agreement (MoAs) between hospitals. The MoAs specify that patients, following assessment and possible treatment, will be repatriated to their home hospitals. Unless patients are repatriated, beds in the host hospital will be used that could be taken up by local patients.

The floor nurse explained to me how a patient's enrolment in a drug trial interfered with this process of repatriation. One of her primary jobs, as she describes it, is to facilitate transfers back to their home hospitals. She describes how she originally believed that being sent to a regional centre would be 'in the patients' best interests'. The intent is to allow them to receive testing and other care not available through their community hospital, including rt-PA, before they are sent back to their home hospital. As she explains, the patient's involvement in research studies delays this process. She said:

> I thought the idea of [providing] 24 hours rt was an excellent idea and it really was in the patients' best interest. Even if there wasn't a bed available. I thought it was, but [in] my experience, it's not working anymore. Because there are now several studies that we're involved with here that keep patients for five days post–rt-PA, even if they're bypass patients, so I can't remember the last person I sent back from bypass.

For this nurse, caring for bypass patients who remain in beds for five days post-rt-PA solely because they are involved in research studies is not in the patient's best interests.[1] In a sense, part of the work being done at the hospital is the production of evidence. It becomes part of the day-to-day work performed by clinicians and affects their practice, as the nurse describes above. It is assumed that the production of this evidence will benefit patient care. A closer empirical examination reveals that this is not always the case. As the floor nurse explains to me, above, the bypassed patients are not being repatriated to their home hospitals because they are participating in 'several studies'.

This also affects the work that physicians do. For example, one community physician explained to me that he didn't mind being on call while he was in the community because 'to be truthful, I was running a clinical trial, so my way of capturing every patient was to tell the emergency room docs and nurses as soon as a stroke comes in, call me on the phone and then I'll decide if it's appropriate or not'. In this instance, the physician's decision to make herself or himself available to be on call for any potential stroke patients is partially related to his involvement in a clinical trial. He says that he doesn't mind being on call because then he can screen patients for participation in his trial.

Participating in clinical trials is a way of maintaining or increasing a physician's academic status. Increasingly, physicians working in academic health centres are called upon to train in Master's programmes, usually in epidemiology, so that they can become clinician-scientists. Few have studied how this affects their working conditions or their ability to provide care for their patients. The assumption remains that research will lead to increasingly better treatments and interventions. But it may also reduce the hours a physician is available to provide direct patient care.

In the EBM and KT literature, physician decision-making is sometimes theorized as being the result of their personal experiences of any given treatment (Gabbay & le May, 2006). So, for example, if they have a good experience they will continue to use a treatment; however, if they have a bad experience, they will not. The physicians I interviewed who were involved in research trials for rt-PA were more likely to advocate its use regardless of their experiences. In the following account, two physicians I spoke with described witnessing the miracle of rt-PA. In the following account, one of the specialists describes his experience:

> I infused the patient within half an hour and the patient began moving his arms, and within an hour he was talking to me. So you know, it was one of these Lazarus phenomenon, and whether it was the rt-PA or not, who knows, the point is that it was such an impressive thing that I fell in love with it. I said, 'Wow, this is the way to go'. So if I had a bad experience I would have been more cautious, but my first case was a Lazarus type of thing. Get up and go, pretty well. He walked out of the hospital with no deficit.

Note the comment, 'whether it was the rt-PA or not, who knows'. The mechanism by which rt-PA resolves ischemic stroke is not as well understood as one might expect. For a certain percentage of strokes, there is no way of knowing if the patient's symptoms would have resolved on their own. Hence, though the physician was unwilling to attribute the resolution to the rt-PA, he 'falls in love' with it. Later, this same specialist went on to have negative experiences. As he described it:

> To the extent that years later I was wondering what I was doing, and sure, I began double guessing myself, not wanting to do it because I had disasters. I had bilateral brain haemorrhages in people whom I felt were ideal candidates, and not just from the site of the stroke bilateral, disastrous, so you know, I've killed probably three to four people with rt-PA since I started giving it in 1996.

Despite 'not wanting to do it because I had disasters', this physician continues to administer rt-PA for acute stroke. He was involved in the trials for rt-PA and works at a specialized centre that delivers this treatment—and so he continues, despite having 'killed probably three to four people'. Another community physician I spoke with references the long-term benefit that rt-PA could provide and acknowledges that it is a benefit he may never witness, but still believes in. He says:

> I've seen the data from the studies, and there's not a lot of magic in that, but to me it just raises the whole issue of disability, of later disability. With the drug you might make a 50 per cent recovery. Without the drug you might make a 30 per cent recovery; well that's a big difference to a person's life even though I might not see that. I can't appreciate it at the bedside whether it's done good or not.

This physician was one of the few who referenced the fact that the main effect of rt-PA in the original National Institute of Neurological Disorders and Stroke (NINDS) Trial could only be observed at three months. No scientific evidence produced through RCTs supports the observation of the Lazarus Effect. It is interesting that it continues to play such a large role in public promotion of rt-PA and also in physician conversations.

In the accounts provided above, the physician's experience does not explain their treatment decisions. Yet most doctors predicted that, for *other* physicians, having an early bad experience could affect your decision to treat with rt-PA in the future. This echoes the professional discourse of KT in which individual-level explanations are used to explain variation in physician practice. For example, one specialist said:

> I think you just have to have one bad bleed and it colours your whole use of things, you know. A young man of 56 that was a diabetic, he came in and he fit the bill very nicely, and he had a moderately severe deficit. He was a good candidate for it and unfortunately he bled [after receiving rt-PA]. But he had a very high sugar at the time and it wasn't completely controlled, so we recognized that as an adverse feature to his case. But it was a sad one because he was a young man. Once you have a big bad bleed the chances are you're going to go to the happy hunting ground, as we say.

Again, this 'one bad bleed' did not prevent this physician from continuing to deliver this treatment. He is, however, postulating that a negative experience might affect *someone else's* treatment decisions when he says 'I think you just have to have one bad bleed and it colours your whole use of things'. Another specialist claims that he bases his decisions on the scientific evidence. As he describes it, 'I understand that the outcomes are worse without it, so I'm willing to impose on the patient the small risk of haemorrhage for the large benefit of results. It's just a trade-off issue'. This same specialist, however, also believes that other non-specialists will not understand and so will be more strongly influenced by their negative experiences.

In situated practice, the experience of delivering rt-PA for acute stroke may or may not fit the experiences reported from the original NINDS trial. The results can be positive but not necessarily attributable to rt-PA; they may be positive but not necessarily observed, and they may be negative but not prevent the physician from using it again. The contradictory outcomes from delivering rt-PA for acute stroke are well highlighted in the following account by a physician who worked in the community:

> And I've had one other case that I can remember well of a patient that presented with a brain stem stroke that we thrombolysed and who had complete resolution of symptoms, remarkable resolution and 24 hours later … he died.

The basic goal of the Ontario Stroke Strategy (OSS) was to improve patient access to best practice care across the continuum. However, as noted, the strategy did arise from advancements for an acute care intervention. In this chapter, I consider how the centrality of acute care in the development of the Ontario Stroke Strategy has affected the rest of the continuum, especially since RCTs cannot be as easily conducted in most sectors for reasons of funding or design.

In the course of my work establishing District Stroke Centres I began to hear, from nurses and physiotherapists, what they considered to be a significant and relative lack of resources provided for stroke rehabilitation and long-term care. At scientific conferences, rehabilitation and prevention are called allied health and are segregated with nursing into less well-attended sessions. I also learned that with proper care, such as the reduction of blood pressure, approximately 80 per cent of all strokes may be preventable (Beaglehole, 2001).

Other critical scholars have written about the nature of the evidence that is produced through meta-analyses of RCTs, which is widely considered by the medical and scientific communities to be the gold standard of research evidence. As previously mentioned, RCTs favour both technology and pharmaceutical interventions. It is difficult to get gold standard evidence about poverty and health, for example, or prevention (Petticrew, 2007). As one researcher noted, 'In an era of competing priorities, decisions to fund clinical research are also decisions not to fund other things' (Gupta, 2003, p. 118). This is particularly important for stroke care, which is both preventable and for which the majority of patients will require some form of rehabilitation.

All the physicians I spoke with expressed how important primary and secondary prevention was in relation to stroke care. They saw this as the place to invest money and resources. This was true for both specialists and community physicians. In the following account, a community physician compares prevention to rt-PA, saying, 'Prevention, I guess, is the main issue more than anything because that's the thing we can do something about. Most of the other things you know, like rt-PA, I don't want to belittle it too much, but there's a certain amount of band-aid to it'. Many others echoed the sentiment that rt-PA was a useful but insufficient response to stroke. One specialist said, 'Well, you know, rt-PA is all I have to offer people in the emergency room, and I think it's important to realize that it's just a start and it's not the end. Because God forbid, if the best we've got to offer people is thrombolysis, that doesn't pump me up at all'. He went on to sum it up this way:

[Prevention is] where you're ultimately going to have your biggest effect, although it's probably not really sexy or appealing to do it. It's easy to intervene with somebody in the emergency room ... but I think there's a bigger question and they've got to address the issue of primary prevention. That goes across diabetes management, endocrinology, internal medicine, cardiology, neurology, across the board.

In a period of health care reform in which strong emphasis is put on controlling costs, the lack of resources going into stroke prevention is puzzling. One study found that while it would be difficult to calculate specific estimates, improving stroke prevention would yield substantial benefits, including the reduction of costs (Goldstein, 2008). A community physician said, 'I think it's what the province should be doing; it should be saying, boy, we can save millions of dollars by preventing strokes, we should be investigating it, finding out how to do it better'.

As noted, primary prevention does not lend itself to pharmaceutical or technological interventions that can be subjected to an RCT. This has been summed up by the statement, 'it takes a lot of gold to meet the gold standard of the clinical trial' (Hess, 1998, p. 17). Or, As Timmermans and Berg (2003) note:

> The reliance on what is currently considered the 'best' evidence, findings validated with randomized clinical trials, often remains out of reach for emerging medical professionals and medical practices at the health care periphery. Randomized clinical trials are labor intensive and expensive to run, they are tailored to particular patient populations [often not those regularly encountered in primary care, such as children and elderly patients], and do not apply easily to all clinical situations. How, for example, does one design a clinical trial for 'cultural competency'? (p. 93)

The institutional explanations for why more resources do not go into prevention are rarely explored. Instead, the tendency to apply psychological or individual-level theories to explain physician behaviour permeates the EBM and KT literature (Alderson, 1998; Eccles et al., 2007). These explanations came up time and again in my discussions with physicians as well. For instance, one family physician I interviewed spoke in detail about how many new family physicians, in his opinion, did not want to deal with elderly patients as they were too time-consuming. He told me:

> Many family doctors now might choose to do just sports medicine. There's nothing wrong with this, but some will—and I think this is unethical—set up shop three floors up, no elevators, make no house calls. Guess what happens? They don't get any geriatrics.

When I ask if he thinks they are doing this on purpose, he responds, 'Of course they are, of course they are. And that's almost unethical; it's just on the edge'.

When I query this physician about why new family doctors don't want to treat elderly patients, he explains:

> Because they're a lot of care. You have to sort of like older people, and admittedly some people aren't too fussy about that. It's just a personality thing. They are not as lucrative; we're not paid as well for geriatrics. You can't see four elderly people in 20 minutes. You can see four ears in

20 minutes. So there's some cruelty to that. So since all strokes are 50 plus [i.e., in age], and most of them are even older, they sort of fit into that.

The idea that it is a 'personality thing' is a persistent theme in the KT discourse and of course stands in contrast to the issue of payment, which is structural and also alluded to in this passage. As previously noted, individual-level explanations abound, and there is a tendency for older physicians to speak about the attitudes of younger physicians, for example, or for specialists to theorize about family physicians. These types of explanations were also provided by the physicians I spoke with. Some physicians felt that more education was required in the community in order to deliver more effective prevention care. For example, one specialist at an urban teaching hospital said:

> I think there's a tremendous amount of education required in the community to prevent stroke. I think this is really the issue because the therapies for stroke are still fairly primitive. And it's better than it was, we no longer put patients on [i.e., in] the back wards and let them aspirate; you know, we have very good stroke protocols, we've made progress. Every patient who is admitted to our hospital now goes to the unit and is monitored and has an aspiration protocol, but it's just that we simply can't manage the numbers that we have in [our area].

In this explanation, an implicit assumption is made that education rather than resources are required to prevent stroke. In addition, despite their recognition of the need for prevention, physicians, especially stroke specialists, were less certain of *who* should deliver prevention services. This parallels the debate around who should deliver acute care interventions. Both specialists and community physicians thought that no one had the time or resources to practise prevention, either primary or secondary. As one specialist said, 'A neurologist intervenes with people with TIAs or stroke, so we're already talking about secondary prevention. You don't have enough neurologists to deal with primary intervention. The GPs and internists out there don't do it'.

It becomes clear in these accounts that not only are physicians not *a* homogenous group, but also they seem to have very little knowledge of what their colleagues do or don't do by way of providing care. There is a clear lack of consensus as to who should be delivering primary or secondary prevention. While everyone acknowledges its importance, no one seems to be linked to producing evidence for it. Little by way of text or discourse formally links physicians who practise prevention (i.e., family physicians) with specialists, and nothing that links either with prevention. Prevention strategies are simply rarely funded for, or eligible for, an RCT. This results in a situation where there is little best practice evidence to support prevention.

Most attribute gaps in health care delivery at the primary level to how busy the primary care physicians are (Tremblay et al., 2004). This has become such an assumed convention in popular thought that it is rarely empirically examined. One specialist told me, 'My impression here is that the family physicians are very busy. I don't really think the GPs in the community can do it all'. Other physicians had similar experiences, citing lack of time and resources to do adequate follow-up with patients as the following account by a community physician highlights:

> No, we don't do any [prevention work]. I don't see patients back to do this. They get the smoking and the cholesterol lecture as part of the consult, but I don't bring them back as I would if I had more time to sit them down and 'let's discuss for the next 30 minutes your risk factors and how we might intervene'. That's all given, or the treadmill experience or the single consult experience, but I rarely invite patients back for a follow-up to do this, and I think this is where we're failing.

The importance that everyone places on prevention is a clear moment of disjuncture from the actual resources that go into prevention. I would suggest that since prevention is not part of the production machine of evidence-based medicine, it cannot enter into the EBM discourse. Thus it cannot enter into practice. Within the KT discourse, other reasons are provided for why prevention is not more widely practised, and these tend to centre on how busy primary care physicians are.

## DEBATING THE EVIDENCE

Eventually I began to wonder how much physicians in the community actually disagreed with the evidence for rt-PA. As noted earlier, the variation rate in the use of rt-PA across hospitals and regions has often been addressed in the literature as a debate about the evidence. For example, an emergency physician writing in the *Western Journal of Medicine* noted that an intervention is only beneficial if it can be practised without harm outside of the 'idealized setting of an expert-based study' (Hoffman, 2000, p. 149). He claims that there is an 'enormous propaganda machine pushing the exciting new fashion of thrombolytic therapy for acute ischemic stroke' but believes there is good and even 'overwhelming' reasons to question its 'effectiveness' (p. 149). For Hoffman, the only 'realistic effectiveness study' was a trial that took place within an actual community setting, Cleveland, rather than through the idealized world of the clinical trial. In the Cleveland study, many patients died unnecessarily, as the community physicians were unable to safely deliver rt-PA. The study was quickly halted. However, resources were devoted to improving the education and training of physicians and the studies resumed, eventually resulting in better patient outcomes. The impact of these types of studies on patients and their families is not recounted anywhere; the patient experience is completely erased as science is tested in real-life hospital settings.

Writing at a different time in the same journal, another emergency medicine physician cites a different study, STARS, in order to claim the benefit of rt-PA. He argues that 'coordinated stroke protocols can reduce such hemorrhage rates while also reducing treatment times and protocol violations' (Robinson, 2000, p. 148). He does not question the ability within the community hospital setting to develop a highly specialized stroke team.

Through these debates the curious reductionist character of medical knowledge and scientific knowledge are revealed. The official accounts of the benefit of a particular treatment have smoothed over these debates as they are written into practice guidelines or become protocols used within hospitals.

By the time I was interviewing physicians, the Ontario Stroke Strategy was several years into its development. I began to wonder to what extent the arguments taking place textually in leading science journals were echoed by physicians in the field. None of the physicians I spoke with ever argued against the evidence for rt-PA. As noted, some of them had often been involved in the original trials associated with rt-PA, and they were the same physicians who promoted its use. One specialist saw it this way:

We were clearly looking for something in stroke and pretty desperate. It's hard to keep writing consultation notes about stroke; we're looking for something new, something you can tell the patients, the people that something has changed, maybe you should consider revising your ideas about treating them on back boards, here's some new stuff, here's something that we can do, Aspirin, drugs, here's something about Statin. Here's a trial, a Progress trial, and maybe that combination would help them preventative. So I think you provide them with some of the excitement that you feel yourself about practice.

Studies looking at physician use of evidence in decision-making have assumed that all physicians participate in evidence debates. I asked the physicians directly how they kept up with the evidence. Some of their answers were surprising. Clearly their decisions are based on more than just appraisal of evidence in journals based on RCTs, as in the following account of how a community physician 'keeps up' with the evidence:

> Poorly. I mean, it's a combination of things. You cannot do it one way. This is not—it's probably heresy in—like, I'm eccentric, but I get a lot of information from the drug reps ... naturally in a teaching hospital you go to rounds and you hear people at the forefront of whatever they are doing, and you can ask them. You can always go next door and say, 'Have you heard about this or do you know about this?' And they explain it to you; so teaching centres are great for that. But when you're in the community, you're depending on publications, on going to rounds if you have the time, like I always came to rounds here, you know, over the years to keep myself informed. You go to conferences, some of the CMEs [Continuing Medical Education] that the reps put together and again are biased but informative, and if you have any degree of critical thinking, you can get from that what you need.

This physician tells me that much of the evidence he reads is 'from drug reps'. That is one of the ways in which he keeps up with the evidence. Despite his assertion that this is 'heresy', this tendency has been noted by others, and the issue of determining the relationship between drug companies and clinical decision-making is controversial (Brennan et al., 2006; Dana & Loewenstein, 2003). What I would like to draw attention to in this account is the nature of evidence to which he refers. The evidence, for him, is clearly related to pharmaceutical trials, underscoring the taken-for-granted character of EBM best practices as pharmaceutical or technological interventions. He also reports that it is difficult to keep up with all the growing evidence.

He also reports that it is difficult to keep up with all the growing evidence. Researchers have commented on the growing accumulation of evidence (Graham et al., 2006) and how the sheer volume of it makes it difficult, if not impossible, for practitioners to keep up with studies as they are produced. As one community physician told me as he raised his hand and sighed, 'Take a look around; I mean, I've got piles of stuff everywhere, and yes, it's a huge problem'.

These expressions of frustration about keeping up contradict the idea of a debate between the emergency room physicians and the stroke specialists in terms of their appraisal of the evidence for acute stroke therapy. The discourse of evidence-based medicine that is so familiar to the stroke specialists is distant from the work of the community physician. They try to keep up but are not linked to the production of evidence and thus are not part of the conversations taking place. Reading, rather than producing, evidence is part of their everyday working lives.

To summarize then, as I have shown, the majority of treatments that are considered evidence-based best practice are based on clinical trials that take place under idealized conditions. They favour interventions that are pharmaceutical or technological. The OSS was built around the development of an acute stroke intervention and around the principles of EBM. Through this organization, other parts of the continuum became in some sense add-ons and, being less central, were less resourced.

Through this analysis it becomes clear that scientific or medical knowledge erases or dismisses as inferior any other type of knowledge, for instance, the knowledge of the community hospital clinicians. Using the knowledge-to-action model described in Chap. 2, Graham et al. (2006) depict the knowledge creation stage of KT as a funnel:

> The knowledge funnel represents knowledge creation and consists of the major types of knowledge or research that exist and can be used in health care ... As knowledge moves through the funnel, it becomes more distilled and refined and presumably more useful to stakeholders. Another analogy would be to think of the research being sifted through filters at each phase so that, in the end, only the most valid and useful knowledge is left. (p. 18)

In this description, knowledge is reified and abstracted. It exists and can be 'used'. It moves through a fictional funnel, becoming increasingly refined and therefore more useful to abstract stakeholders. It is sifted until 'only the most valid and useful knowledge is left'. But who does the sifting? Who determines its usefulness to stakeholders? Who in fact determines who the stakeholders are?

The notion of the physician problem is generated within a discourse that favours interventions developed in settings with academic specialists but often aimed towards those working in the community settings. In addition, the organization of the Ontario Stroke Strategy provides a link between the work of the Heart and Stroke Foundation of Ontario (HSFO), the Ministry of Health and Long-Term Care (MoHLTC) and academic physicians. Through the academic physicians, this may also link the work of the pharmaceutical industry with the work of the university, although this would require further study. I would like to suggest that promoting rt-PA did seem to allow physicians to recruit more patients for their studies. Promoting rt-PA also becomes important to the aims of the HSFO, a charitable foundation which relies on donations, as outlined in Chap. 2. The acceptance and promotion of rt-PA for acute stroke by the HSFO and MoHLTC legitimize and neutralize the interests of pharmaceutical companies, albeit unintentionally. Innovation, it would seem, does not just improve the health of Canadians, as is frequently claimed. It would appear that the direction of benefit may also run along the same lines as the direction of innovation.

## NOTE

1. Rankin and Campbell (2006) have described how the practice of setting and monitoring patient's length of stay as a key indicator of hospital performance has led to some staff viewing patients as bed blockers.

## REFERENCES

Alderson, P. (1998). Theories in health care and research: The importance of theories in health care. *British Medical Journal, 317*, 1007–1010.

Beaglehole, R. (2001). Global cardiovascular disease prevention: Time to get serious. *Lancet, 358*, 661–663.

Brennan, T. A., Rothman, D. J., Blank, L., Blumenthal, D., Chimonas, S. C., Cohen, J. J., et al. (2006). Health industry practices that create conflicts of interest: A policy proposal for academic medical centers. *Journal of the American Medical Association, 295*, 429–433.

Dana, J., & Loewenstein, G. (2003). A social science perspective on gifts to physicians from industry. *Journal of the American Medical Association, 290*, 252–255.

Eccles, M. P., Grimshaw, J. M., Johnston, M., Steen, N., Pitts, N. B., Thomas, R., et al. (2007). Applying psychological theories to evidence-based clinical practice: Identifying factors predictive of managing upper respiratory tract infections with antibiotics. *Journal of Implementation Science, 2*, 26.

Gabbay, J., & le May, A. (2006). Evidence based guidelines or collectively constructed mindlines? Ethnographic study of knowledge management in primary care. *British Medical Journal, 329*, 1013.

Goldstein, L. B. (2008). How much can be gained by more systematic prevention of stroke? *International Journal of Stroke, 3*(4), 266–271.

Graham, I., Logan, J., Harrison, M. B., Straus, S. E., Tetroe, J., Caswell, W., et al. (2006). Lost in translation: Time for a map? *Journal of Continuing Education in the Health Professions, 26*, 13–24.

Gupta, M. (2003). A critical appraisal of evidence-based medicine: Some ethical considerations. *Journal of Evaluation in Clinical Practice, 9*, 111–121.

Hess, D. (1998). *Can bacteria cause cancer? Alternative medicine confronts big science.* New York: New York University Press.

Hoffman, J. (2000). And just what is the emperor of stroke wearing? *Western Journal of Medicine, 174*, 149–150.

Lambert, H. (2005). Accounting for EBM: Notions of evidence in medicine. *Social Science & Medicine, 62*, 2633–2645.

Petticrew, M. (2007). More research needed: Plugging gaps in the evidence base on health inequalities. *European Journal of Public Health, 17*, 411–413. https://doi.org/10.1093/eurpub/ckm094

Rankin, J. M., & Campbell, M. L. (2006). *Managing to nurse: Inside Canada's health care reform.* Toronto, ON: University of Toronto Press.

Robinson, D. (2000). Thrombolytics in stroke: Whose risk is it anyway? *Western Journal of Medicine, 173*, 148–149.

Timmermans, S., & Berg, M. (2003). *The gold standard: The challenge of evidence-based medicine and standardization in health care.* Philadelphia: Temple University Press.

Tremblay, G. J. L., Drouin, D., Parker, J., Monette, C., Cote, D. F., & Reid, R. D. (2004). The Canadian Cardiovascular Society and knowledge translation: Turning evidence into best practice. *Canadian Journal of Cardiology, 20*, 1195–1198.

# CHAPTER 5

# Variations in the Implementation of Best Practice: From Academic Hospital to Community Settings

The first physician I interviewed from a Regional Stroke Centre (RSC) is a neurologist. He is part of a large, tertiary care urban teaching hospital and practices in the ideal setting presupposed in the original National Institute of Neurological Disorders and Stroke Trial for thrombolytic therapy (rt-PA). We are sitting in a small musty library in the hospital with the walls lined with shelves of medical journals and stacks of books piled on the floor. It's quiet and far away from the hospital floor where care is delivered. Just outside the window is the helicopter pad where some of the patients arrive by air ambulance. The specialist will be paged several times during our conversation, and I will soon come to recognize this as part and parcel of every interview with a physician that I will do, underscoring for me how busy and unpredictable clinical life is and not lending itself readily to standardization. Various codes will be called at fairly frequent intervals, denoting different levels of response that are required. Nevertheless, the specialist is polite and patiently willing to answer my questions.

As we begin, I ask him to take me through an account of delivering rt-PA for acute stroke. He chooses a case and then, leaving out any patient detail, describes the process of care. Within health care, every patient is turned into a case by a set of textual practices that erases his or her experiences and subordinates them to the categories artificially produced. The specialist is describing how he makes the decision about whether or not to

© The Author(s) 2020
F. Webster, *The Social Organization of Best Practice*,
https://doi.org/10.1007/978-3-030-43165-5_5

treat this case with rt-PA. In this first passage, he references a particular patient he recently treated:

> It's kind of interesting. There were multiple different sorts of novel techniques, things we did, and we probably wouldn't have done elsewhere. But essentially they called me. I was on call. [I asked] several questions to make sure, to rule out things. I would not give rt-PA [without ruling out] things like haemorrhage and severe injury or seizures. He had none of those.

In this account, the physician talks about making decisions autonomously. He discusses the conditions under which he would give or not give rt-PA. He also makes reference to the fact that he was on call when he was contacted about the patient. This is a critical component of being able to deliver this service. With few specialists working in the community, there are also fewer physicians with whom to share call. One specialist may have to be on call several days a week, with enormous impact on their personal lives and their levels of fatigue.

The account continues. The specialist notes casually that he arranged to have the patient airlifted by helicopter. He then examines the patient again. As he recounts it, 'I examined him; he had effectively a moderately severe stroke. And then I gave him [the drug] in the emergency room'. It is notable that the physician refers to the fact that he 'gave him' the actual drug in the emergency room. As I will show later, the nurse and not the physician normally does this, a small example of how people are invisible in professional accounts of work. The specialist continues to tell me how he had felt confident with his decision. He explained, 'I had called all the appropriate people, [such as] the radiologist, to actively get them to come in and set up the angiographic suite for the direct rt-PA'.

This specialist emphasizes to me that he always uses a computed tomography (CT) scan. In response to my question as to whether or not he undertook a CT scan in this case, the specialist responds emphatically,

> Always, always, always. CT, always, there's no doubt. I will do three CTs, a CT is like basic. It's probably even more important than my neurological examination. It's key, and it provides so much information, so definitely.

In the ideal setting of the Academic Health Sciences Centre, a CT scan is readily available. The specialist can do 'three CTs' if necessary. In the community setting, even when a hospital has a CT scanner, there may be heavy demands on it or 'no radiologist around' to interpret the results.

Once the patient has been deemed eligible for treatment, rt-PA must then be given. The following is a description by a specialist working in a large urban teaching hospital about the actual process of administering rt-PA. This response is in answer to my question, 'Is giving rt-PA time-consuming?'

> Yes, it is, because first you have to have a fairly well-organized team that responds appropriately and effectively and quickly. So you have to be available and be able to sort of leave the ER for 15 to 20 minutes and then, once they arrive and if you're going to give rt-PA, then they're admitted for the next 3 to 4 hours. You're doing things, luckily, and you go down and get the patient set up for admission, make sure all the blood work is done [and that] the IV is in the appropriate space. You're keeping an eye constantly on the patient, clinically making sure there hasn't been any change, different things.

In this account, a 'fairly well-organized team' is in place that allows the specialist to respond appropriately and effectively. For this specialist, the presence and availability of this team is a taken-for-granted reality. How this gets acted out in the various situated practices is quite different, such as when a stroke specialist is not available to coordinate all these different activities.

The professional discourse of this account hides the presence of many others involved in the delivery of this care. As previously noted in Chap. 2, Smith identifies two aspects of what she refers to as 'work knowledges' (Smith, 2005, p. 151). The first of these is a person's experience of what they do, think and feel. The second is the 'implicit or explicit coordination of his or her work with the work of others' (2005, p. 151). Citing the example of an interview she did with a steelworker, Smith notes that in his account there were 'unexplicated presences'. She says,

> We might think of this aspect of people's experiential accounts of their work as doors through which the ethnographer may go to open up further resources of knowledge from those at work on the other side of a particular story. Of special importance ... are the texts that enter into the organization of people's work and how the text coordinates different work processes. Here are often to be found the key linkages between one person's work and that of others. (2005, 161)

Through my observation, a door was opened through which I began to see 'those at work on the other side of a particular story'.

## OBSERVATIONS

In March 2005, I was having coffee with a specialist in the hospital cafeteria when he received a page from a nurse in emergency that a stroke patient arrived who might be eligible for rt-PA. He and I walk quickly down to the emergency department, through a route I've never taken before, at the back of the hospital that leads us straight into one of the examining rooms in the emergency department. On the way down, the specialist is explaining to me what he knows about this patient from the page. Someone, presumably a nurse already in the emergency department, has already gathered some information. The patient, who I will refer to as Lucy, is 80 years old and has come from another town. Lucy was not sent to her home hospital, as it could not administer rt-PA; as noted in Chap. 4, this is referred to as a bypass. Her stroke onset was 9:00 a.m., so within the three-hour window. The specialist says he will need to decide if she is an eligible patient or one at risk for haemorrhage, which he refers to as a bleed. He also mentions that these strokes are generally severe in order for others to recognize them.

We walk into the examining room where a woman is lying quietly in a bed. She looks peaceful and younger than my image of an 80-year-old woman. She also looks well to me; there is nothing about her that strikes me as unusual.

The specialist begins speaking to the two nurses who are already in the room and seem to have already begun some of the steps involved in providing care. An emergency department nurse is drawing blood. The other nurse, who seems more senior, tells the physician that the patient is aphasic (can't speak), was weak, couldn't support herself, and that the husband was a witness. The specialist responds, 'So, it's good' (meaning she may be eligible for rt-PA). They also discuss whether or not the woman may have come from a non-English speaking country and if this is affecting her lack of response to questions. The specialist points out that the woman's weakness is already resolving. He says, 'See how she puts her legs crossed; she can't do this if she's paraplegic'.

A study nurse then arrives and tries to talk to the patient. This nurse is a trained registered nurse (RN) whose role in the hospital is to manage clinical trials. She rearranges the woman's air tube and talks to the emergency department nurse. It looks to me as if Lucy smiled at her, but later I'll notice that this is her response to everything. The study nurse asks the nurse if the patient is on aspirin—yes.

The specialist then receives a page from a stroke fellow from within the hospital. He picks up the phone in the treatment room. Stroke fellows are neurologists who are completing a two-year research or clinical fellowship. The fellow is paging with a research question about a research database he is setting up. The specialist indicates that he is in emergency and will have to call him back.

The specialist then approaches Lucy. He asks her to smile, stick out her tongue and asks, 'How old are you?' He suggests some ages—60? 70? 80? She does not respond. This is when I begin to notice that indeed something is wrong. The study nurse and the specialist begin ranking the severity of the woman's deficits using the National Institutes of Health (NIH) Stroke Scale.[1] They are sharing the same plastic card and go through the questions together and come up with a number—10. But there are still other tests to be performed.

The study nurse is then paged out of the room. The emergency department nurse picks up the telephone and asks to book a CT scan. She has taken the woman's blood pressure and reports that it is high. The study nurse comes back in the room and lightly pricks both sides of the patient's face with what appears to be a simple, silver pin. The specialist says 'Do her leg, it might be 11. Her one leg is weak, so then, OK for our study, score her a 12'. These actions being performed by the study nurse, then, are to determine the patient's eligibility for a drug study.

The more senior nurse leaves the room and another arrives. I do not know who the new nurse is. The new nurse says that the woman is 86 years old. The specialist fills out a form called a Consultant's Report. As he does this, the new nurse telephones the patient's husband. She tells the specialist that the person with Lucy in the morning had been her friend, not her husband. The specialist then takes the phone and speaks to the husband. He says, 'Do you know what a stroke is? A stroke is caused by a blockage in the artery. When part of the brain dies, it causes symptoms. It seems like your wife is having a stroke'. The study nurse then takes the phone and speaks to the husband, asking him for his consent to include Lucy in the study she is conducting for the physician.

A social worker then arrives and announces that the patient's daughter is on the telephone line for the specialist to speak with. In the meantime, the study nurse has telephoned the patient's son, on another line, to ask for consent for her study. The specialist confirms with the daughter that the patient was OK when she woke up this morning. The specialist asks, 'Did she speak to you? Do you live together?' It is critical to determine the time when the patient was 'last seen well' given the three-hour time window in which rt-PA can be administered.

The paramedics then come into the room briefly. They don't speak, except to say hello to the staff, look around and then leave. I am told that they will now wait to see if the patient needs to be transported back to her home hospital.[2] At 9:50 a.m. an unidentified person comes to take the patient for a CT scan. This entire process in the emergency room has been quick and hectic.

Both the specialist and the study nurse end their respective telephone calls. The two emergency department nurses begin getting the room ready for the administration of rt-PA, setting up IV drips and checking for the actual drug. The study nurse reports that the son is on his way into the hospital. She will give him more information about Lucy when he arrives. Her son has described his mother as 'independent' and 'stubborn'. Interestingly, I am told that this information will be used by the team to assess what the patient's preference might have been in terms of receiving treatment. The specialist says that he found out that the patient was with a friend by chance. 'He's an old friend as well' and confirms that Lucy was well upon waking. The specialist then begins filling out notes in his Consultant's Report.

The study nurse, the emergency department nurse, the specialist and I walk to the back elevator. The specialist is still writing notes. He says, 'So the son will be in his 70s', and the study nurse replies, '68'. The specialist explains that he doesn't need official consent but will explain rt-PA to the family. The study nurse does need consent for the study she is coordinating for the physician. The study nurse provides information for this to the emergency department nurse who is filling out the consent form.

We arrive at the CT scan department where another patient's scan is in progress and sit waiting in a small room beside the scanner with two large screens upon which to view the CT scans. The specialist continues to write up notes for his Consultant's Report. Lucy is taken in for her scan by a technician. The technician goes into the scan room and says, 'Hold still'. Another nurse arrives so we are five in a small room. The nurses are discussing the weather; the specialist asks what the date is; a nurse calls to make an appointment for a haircut.

Within a very short time, the specialist is reading the scans that are now up on the screen. He wonders out loud if he's looking at an old stroke. He also comments that the scan is not clear because Lucy kept moving. She had tilted her head and, because she couldn't respond to directions, they couldn't communicate with her to remain still. The specialist says, 'This is the brain of an 80-year-old woman'. But he finds it 'hard to say' about her current stroke and so pages a senior consultant. We are also told by one of the nurses arriving to the room that the son has now arrived. The specialist says out loud, 'Son is here by 11:30, two hours after onset, so we still have time'.

Someone tells the specialist that Lucy's blood pressure is a bit high. The study nurse indicates that she is being treated for high blood pressure. The nurse is waiting for a list of medications from Lucy's pharmacy to be faxed over from another town. At 10:58 a.m. Lucy is wheeled back to the treatment room in emergency by a staff person. We remain in the scanner room. The telephone rings; it is the consultant answering the specialist's page. The specialist recounts to him the following information, quickly and without pausing:

> Bypass protocol, half hour ago
> Woke up this a.m. fine
> 9:30 or 9:15
> Had breakfast
> [Study Nurse interjects: 'We should look at the ambulance record; I'll get it when we go downstairs']
> Global aphasic, alert
> NIH scale 11 or 12
> Study is here
> Son on his way, within 20 minutes
> Have CT scan that is in front of me
> High blood pressure and prior stroke—recovered except for problem with writing
> Waiting for list of meds
> Blood pressure of 185/114—10 minutes ago
> Independent—does her own cooking
> She [i.e., the patient] has gone back down to emergency

The specialist hangs up and the consultant is then on his way to the CT scanner. He arrives within minutes. Everyone who is in the room is staring at the scans of Lucy's brain. I try to see if I can visibly discern anything, but I cannot. The consultant says:

No bleed
Signs of more than one infarct [stroke]
Look for acute ischemic changes
Hard to say because she's turning her head
Older brain with fragile vessels
10–15 per cent chance of bleeding
Could worsen—won't recover

A nurse informs both the consultant and the specialist that the neuro-radiologist has the scan now. I assume this has been sent to him electronically, as he is not in the room with us. The study nurse, the specialist, the consultant and I all walk out of the scanner room and back to the emergency room. At the elevators, the consultant says, 'I'm not comfortable with you seeing a patient', and asks me to leave. The specialist comes back down later to tell me that they have decided not to give Lucy rt-PA after the neuroradiologist had seen the scan.

Both these accounts describe the administration of rt-PA by stroke specialists in Regional Stroke Centres. They represent what can be offered in an ideal setting. This is not to suggest that problems do not arise in these settings; however, the treatment of rt-PA was designed within and tested in these settings in which a high degree of technology and human resources are available. The degree of social coordination within the three-hour time frame is quite remarkable with a strikingly high number of people involved. Within one hour during my observation, the procedure has involved three trained nurses, two paramedics, a neurologist, a stroke consultant, unidentified staff who have transported the patient to and from the emergency room, pharmacy staff, a technician who operates the CT scanner and a neuroradiologist. An advanced practice nurse has assisted the physician in determining the severity of the patient's stroke; several nurses have been involved in obtaining relevant clinical information from family members and friends.

But what happens in other centres? What assumptions underlie this account, assumptions that do not occur in the situated practice of the community setting? I draw upon the accounts provided by the physicians, other clinicians, family and patients in order to proceed step-by-step through the process of delivering acute stroke care. In doing so, I begin to uncover the disjuncture between the assumptions of evidence-based medicine (EBM) and the local actualities of its translation into practice.

In the following account, a nurse describes a terrible experience she had with a patient afflicted by stroke within a community hospital:

> We did have a gentleman who had a stroke, who pulled out his [feeding] tube and said, 'No, no, no'. And the nurses felt it was very purposeful that he wanted to die, he wanted the tube out. The family wanted it back in, so he was restrained and an urgent psychiatry consult [was held], and we've now tied down the feeding tube. I mean he's 60. He just wanted obviously to die, and that's not uncommon. And it's hard for the nurses to see that. The doctors will say, 'Well, this person is just depressed from the stroke, if we treat the depression they may feel differently'. I don't know how many times I've heard people say that. He's only 62, and his future is going to be a nursing home. Physicians usually will obviously not want to override the family. You're not going to get them doing that very much in this day and age of suing and legalities, so this gentleman is tied down and fed again, so. He's pulled it out now twice, so he's pretty clear on what he wants.

My point in including this nurse's standpoint is not to argue whether or not stroke patients should be assessed for depression or to discuss the important issue of medically assisted dying. However, I think it illustrates the enormous impact of stroke on patients, their families and the medical staff who provide care. It also highlights the implicit promise of EBM for clinicians as well as patients and makes very clear why the notion of an intervention that can completely reverse stroke damage is so appealing. However, in the example of rt-PA, the reality may not be quite as clear or dramatic as the ideal suggests it might be.

The next section presents the accounts of physicians in both community and District Stroke Centres (DSCs) as they go about 'deciding' whether or not to treat acute stroke patients with rt-PA. I then discuss the invisible social relations underpinning and making possible the work that is being described. Writing about mainstream sociology, Smith makes the observation that in theory and in the attempt to be 'objective', people and activities 'disappear from view' (Smith, 2005). In the physician accounts provided in the next section, many others, who were absent in the formal texts of stroke best practices, suddenly appear into view.

## Identification of Stroke

The first step in receiving acute stroke care begins with the patient or an observer. Someone has to be able to recognize a stroke. Even when the patient can recognize a stroke, someone else must be present to confirm the time when the patient was last seen well. However, it is not easy to identify stroke, for even the most attentive observer. For example, with right-sided stroke, patients may be unaware of their own symptoms as damage to the right side of the brain affects the person's perceptions of self and others, as well as muting emotional responses (DiLegge, Fang, Saposnik, & Hachinski, 2005). A right-sided stroke may not always be apparent to others as well for the same reasons. A deficit in emotional awareness may not present as dramatically as, for instance, a drooping arm or facial feature, as is more likely with a left-sided stroke.

This is what happened for Betty, whom I described in Chap. 3. Betty suffered a stroke when she was 60 years old and was unable to recognize her symptoms. She describes for me what happened during her first stroke:

> Actually, I was in my car. Well, I hadn't been having symptoms when I went out in my car. But I had gone to a store, parked my car, and I couldn't get the door open with my left hand, it went quite weak. And I thought, 'What's wrong with me?' I couldn't connect anything. I just thought, 'This is stupid'. So, I put my other hand over, and I opened the car door. I had stopped the car, but I just couldn't get out of the car because I couldn't open it. I opened it with the right hand, and I fell out of the car. But it wasn't as if I couldn't stop myself; I just didn't realize that I was falling out. And I banged my head on the pavement.

In order to increase public awareness of the signs and symptoms of stroke, and to reinforce the idea that stroke constitutes an emergency, the Heart and Stroke Foundation of Ontario launched an education campaign in 1999. Print, radio and television advertising was shown and evaluated across several regions in Ontario in order to determine what method worked best to raise awareness levels of the signs and symptoms of stroke. Earlier survey research had found that a third of respondents aged 45 and older could not name any of the five warning signs. Advertising was created that focused on the five warning signs of stroke. These are the sudden onset of weakness, trouble speaking, vision problems, headache and dizziness. Following the television advertising (which was chosen as the most successful method of communication), the ability to name one or more warning signs increased 27 per cent among those under the age of 65. Interestingly, awareness levels did not change for those 65 and older, although this is the age group most likely to suffer stroke. The Ontario Heart and Stroke advertisements for stroke have continued until the present time.

Despite these 'gains in public awareness', stroke remains difficult both for the public *and for professionals* to accurately diagnose, as real-life situations are more complex than those implied in the advertising. This produces a rather striking disjuncture between both the marketing literature and the debates regarding physician uptake of rt-PA in medical journals in which difficulties with patient and clinician identification of stroke are often glossed over. The following account, by John, a patient's son, describes the difficulty for onlookers in correctly identifying stroke. His 80-year-old mother suffered a stroke while she was at the cottage. Bystanders did not recognize it as such. She was taken to a small community hospital and sent home, still undiagnosed. She was transferred to a Regional Stroke Centre (at the son's urging) where she was diagnosed as having had a stroke. I interviewed the son, John, while his mother was still in a rehabilitation hospital. He tells me:

> She was up at the cottage, and that's where it happened. Earlier in the day, she had gone into town, and I guess that's when it happened. She banged into a couple of cars in the parking lot. Fortunately one of the guys that she hit was kind enough to take her to an ophthalmologist because she was complaining about her vision. They probably saw her as an old lady who's just confused. Yea, she's an old lady driving around in her car, hits a couple people, in the parking lot, gets out, really is sort of confused, doesn't know what's going on, so they probably just assume that she's an old lady. I assume most strokes don't happen around family members. So, yea, that would be kind of hard to catch. I don't know.

In this account, John is reflecting on the Heart and Stroke campaign to help the public identify the signs and symptoms of stroke. At the time Heart and Stroke was heavily promoting that patients and family members should educate themselves to identify the signs of stroke. He points out that the symptoms of stroke may not be as easy to identify as the advertisements suggest. This is the case not only for the public but also for clinicians and other caregivers. Once a stroke has been identified by the patient or onlooker and an ambulance has been called, paramedics must then be able to correctly identify stroke and bypass the patient to the nearest hospital offering acute stroke services. The same difficulties in diagnosing stroke that exist for patients and bystanders also apply to paramedics. In addition, ambulance services are a scarce resource. Ambulances attending one situation are not available to attend another. This is especially an issue in rural and semi-rural areas in which an acute stroke patient must be bypassed from the local hospital to the specialized urban regional centre. Hospital bypass protocols require explicit coordination between hospitals and between the provincial government and the local town or city. Bypassing one hospital for another also involves complex issues of repatriation—when and how the patient, after receiving specialized acute care services, is transported back to the home hospital. In order to improve the paramedics' ability to recognize stroke, a paramedic prompt card was developed through the Ontario Stroke Strategy (OSS).

Once the patient arrives at the hospital, clinicians must then be able to diagnose a stroke. Recall John, the son of the woman who was not accurately identified by onlookers in the parking lot as having had a stroke. John describes in detail how, once they arrive at the community hospital where his mother was first taken, the attending physician did not immediately recognize that his mother had suffered a stroke. He commented: 'They did an assessment of her and didn't think there was anything wrong with her … But it just seems that it was such a basic assessment to me; if they make a poster about it so that every layman knows what the five signs of stroke are, you would think that the doctor [would know]'. Despite John's earlier recognition that the signs and symptoms of stroke may not be as obvious as he had assumed from the advertisements, he still attributes the misdiagnosis of his mother to the failure of the individual physician. He states that it just seems like such a 'basic assessment' to him. However, as I will discuss in the next section, this is not the case.

In summary, these types of differences in local settings are not addressed in the campaigns, which urge the public to treat stroke as an emergency. The general public assumes, of course, that clinicians will be able to accurately diagnose a stroke once they reach hospital. The current emphasis on getting new knowledge into practice—such as the advertising campaigns for acute stroke treatments—may have important considerations for patient expectations of the health care that is available to them. This would be an important area for future study.

## PROBLEMS IN CLINICAL DIAGNOSIS

Many conditions mimic stroke, and often physicians, even specialists, cannot accurately identify one through its clinical signs (Hand, Kwan, Lindley, Dennis, & Wardlaw, 2006). One study quoted in the American Stroke Association (2003) Guidelines for the Early Management of Patients with Ischemic Stroke found that in one series of 821 consecutive patients initially diagnosed with stroke, 13 per cent were later determined to have had other conditions. One of the key clinical tasks in these cases is to take an adequate medical history in order to establish that the stroke onset is less than three hours. This raises the need for stroke specialists to be on hand to deliver care, which contradicts the model of the OSS. As one specialist described it:

> Somebody has to know how to ask the really tough, hard questions. When was this patient normal? You know that this patient was normal, how do you know this stroke happened in the last hour? What was this patient like yesterday? That's the biggest problem; emergency doctors don't ask enough questions. They just take whatever [is] the first answer out of the family's mouth or nurse's mouth or paramedic's mouth. That's my big issue with emergency doctors.

As this account makes clear, specialists do not believe that the provision of stroke paramedic cards or other training provided to community nurses or physicians necessarily provides them with adequate skill to diagnose stroke. This may or may not be the case. However, the issue again refers back to the disjuncture regarding the type of knowledge that is developed, by whom and for whom. The specialist identifies a problem with emergency physicians—that they don't ask enough questions. He is not specific as to how he knows this, or to whom, the physician would ask these hard questions, if not the family, nurse or paramedic.

A family physician delivering care within a community hospital corroborates this view that community physician should not deliver rt-PA for acute stroke. He discusses the lack of access to specialized colleagues in his work setting. As he points out,

> Not everything that presents with neurological symptoms is stroke. This is another issue, and it's quite difficult for us because we don't sometimes have adequate coverage in the emergency room and people who are skilled in making that determination.

So for this physician, not having enough staff in general, and qualified staff in particular, affects his ability to provide rt-PA. Emergency physicians, usually a family physician, who work in the emergency room of a community hospital, often do not have specialized backup at their disposal. They do not have highly specialized colleagues with whom to confer.

## ON CALL ISSUES

In order for a hospital or centre to provide rt-PA for acute stroke, a physician must be on call 24 hours a day. This is particularly an issue in community hospitals or semi-rural District Stroke Centres, where there are few specialists to share the load of being on call. Physician shortages are common in rural and remote areas. Less than 4 per cent of specialists in Canada practise in rural communities of less than 100,000 population areas (Wootton, 2007). This has led to competing priorities of professionals for whom stroke care may not always be a priority. As one specialist who had worked in the community commented:

> There's no compensation for [being on call to provide stroke care]. You are supposed to know that this is going to be a lifelong learning and you're going to try to do it the best you can, but you know, you get involved in so many things and you end up disregarding something else, sometimes your family, sometimes your personal life, sometimes studying.

While funding issues are of concern regionally and provincially, they have a specific flavour in rural communities. Rural physicians face a different scope of practice than their urban colleagues and may be inadequately compensated for their practice (Wootton, 2007). In the following account, a community physician describes how being on call to provide acute stroke services affects his personal life:

> Yea, I have to be there at the bedside; I have to push the plunger on the syringe. I guess the big issue for me is, it's a lifestyle thing. You've got [to] get it to [patients] within three hours. And that's part of the stroke thing; you have to be there as soon as the patient comes, so that you can't go out to a nice restaurant, or shopping if you like, you just have to sit there and be available. And I think a lot of us are pretty resentful about that sort of obligation because it's not funded. If I come in, in the middle of the night, I think I get paid $50. To do that, if I call for an X-ray, or if the X-ray tech

comes in, she gets three hours of pay whether she's there for ten minutes or half an hour.

In this account, what the community physician is describing as a 'lifestyle thing' actually refers to the physician's work conditions. He is also referring to the issue of physician compensation, which is a topic of debate within Canada and other countries, such as the United Kingdom.

In the following account, a physician working in a community setting refers to the on call schedule as 'enslavement'. Even in an urban teaching hospital, with many stroke fellows sharing call, I observed that their schedule was quite overwhelming. They would frequently be called into the hospital many times during the night, interrupting their sleep and their family lives. As one physician described his experiences of working in the community:

> I don't see reluctance on the part of the neurologists except for the enslavement that it produces, so if you are one of two or a single neurologist in a community for a hospital and you agree to do rt-PA, then you have to be available. If you establish that as your standard of treatment in your hospital, then you have to be available and it's enslaving because you cannot go anywhere. You're there all the time.

Recruitment and retention of health care professionals has become an important issue within Ontario. Another physician in a community hospital was particularly vocal about discussing these issues. From his perspective, difficulties in recruiting more staff are directly related to issues of what he terms 'onerous on call schedules':

> The on call is really becoming a huge issue because the younger people, they place lifestyle issues very, very high. They judge a community in terms of how much time they can devote to leisure time activities, and if they're faced with an onerous on call schedule, they're not so tempted to come.

This physician attributes the concern with lifestyle, rather than working conditions, as being an attribute of the younger generation of physicians. As noted earlier, younger clinicians also attribute problems to older physicians. These individual-level explanations based on personality or attitude are representative of explanations within the knowledge translation field that attribute variations in physician practice to personality differences or attitudes rather than looking at what people are actually doing in the work that they perform and how that work is organized.

## Problems with Technology

In 1999, a 35-page survey was sent to 190 hospitals in Ontario inquiring about the spectrum of stroke care (Tu & Porter, 1999). The survey was designed to capture information on many issues, including imaging technology and the readiness of hospitals to administer thrombolytic therapy. This study found that family physicians were the attending physicians at 78 per cent of acute hospitals. At the time, only 59 of 190 hospitals reported that they had a CT scanner. Since that time, more CT scanners have been purchased for hospitals.

However, in addition to having a CT scanner, someone must be available to read the results. A community physician described the lack of a radiologist to read a scan properly in the following account:

> So a lot of time I'm looking at the CT scan myself and trying to read it myself, and I don't know what I'm looking at. I try, I've looked at lots, I've looked at it with the radiologist, I've taken courses, I've looked at video computer pictures. And time and again, the next day I come back and the radiologist looked at things I didn't see. And I remember one case—a guy came in with a pretty major stroke. I looked at his CT scan, I didn't see much; I gave him rt-PA. And then we reviewed with the neuroradiologist in the [city] a little later, and he said, 'Oh gee, bad thing you gave him that rt-PA; look at all the damage on the CT scan'.

I asked, 'Why isn't there a radiologist on call?', and he responded, 'There are no radiologists around'. In this example, a patient had died as a result of being given rt-PA when the CT scan showed that he was not an eligible candidate. Only later, when a radiologist reviewed the scan, was the cause of the patient's death uncovered.

Robert, a retired high school principal, experienced a stroke in a community setting. His experience underscores that even when the technology necessary for identifying stroke is available, it is not always sufficient. Following a CT scan, he describes his experience of the physician's uncertainty.

Well, I waited there for half an hour until the doctor had the results. And he came in and talked to me briefly … I guess they were a little nebulous, and he wasn't totally sure whether I had had a stroke or not. So he suggested that it would be a good idea if I went to the stroke clinic.

Robert's experiences suggest that a CT scan is not always the only, or best, way to diagnose a stroke. Robert goes on to recount how a neurologist in the stroke clinic where he had been sent for further investigation finally diagnosed him through a clinical exam:

[The specialist] said I had had a stroke. He made it very clear, 'Yes, you had a stroke'. He was able to determine that by performing tests [the same tests performed by the original physician]. He just did them for himself and determined that it had been a stroke by comparing muscle strength from the left side of the body to the right. That's basically how he made the determination.

## Patient Preferences

Within the EBM literature, patient preference should be an important part of physician decision-making[3] (Sackett, Richardson, Rosenberg, & Haynes, 1997). Not surprisingly, however, stroke patients are often unable to make a decision for themselves about their treatment, and so the decision falls to the family. This turns out not to be easy for patients or their families, especially given the time-sensitive nature of the decision. One specialist says:

Not being able to make a decision is fairly common because you're giving them all this information [and saying that] this person who you had previously seen perfectly well, if he only had high cholesterol and he was on nothing initially, is now quite ill. So this is a complete shock—this person, no medications, quit smoking a long time ago. This person was perfectly well and is now all of a sudden is having a severe stroke. If we do nothing, he's going to be completely disabled. And you know, it would take me weeks and months to digest that information alone. And we're giving them minutes. And the second element is can we now do something potentially very dangerous, potentially something that might kill them.

Others have noted how meaningless it can be to ask patients to be invited to participate in medical decision-making when they do not understand the discourse of medicine (Rankin & Campbell, 2006). Using the example of a case manager who adopts a 'patient-centred' approach when speaking with a client who is seeking home care, they note that 'without access to adequate information, he [the client] cannot make sensible choices' (p. 95). In the above comment, the specialist is aware that families are being asked to digest information in minutes that it would take him weeks to absorb. To the extent that such decision-making is difficult, the EBM method of taking into account patient preferences cannot be easily applied in the real-world setting. One patient described for me her decision-making process in relation to rt-PA for acute stroke when she was 51 years old. In this example, her treatment was ultimately successful:

> Then they discussed rt-PA and said, 'The way you are right now is the way you're going to be if you don't have it'. And I was paralyzed completely on one side. I couldn't process things. I'm going by what they told me too; [they said that] I would look at them with a vacant look like, 'What are you talking about?' ... They told me that I would be like that, the way I am now; I'd be in a wheelchair, you know probably, or I could have the rt-PA, and it may make a difference. It may not, it might kill me. I remember that, that you could die. I was scared. I thought, 'What do you mean I could die? I can't die', you know. It was terrifying.

In this account, it becomes clear that the patient could not really have made the decision to have rt-PA. She is scared. She describes not being able to process information and explains that bystanders later described her as having a vacant look.

In addition, the EBM method does not take into account the impact on the family of making the 'wrong' decision. Since rt-PA carries a 6 per cent bleed rate, the patient can die of the intervention rather than from the stroke itself. A community physician described for me the impact of this outcome on the family:

> Usually there's a family member making the decision. It's rare that the patient themselves make the decision for rt-PA because they are too sick or they don't understand, whatever. So the family member makes the decision. You're telling this family member, 'Look, you're going to sign this paper because there's a risk that this patient could bleed, and if it happens you [will] feel terrible'. And you see their grief, and you see they're torn. I made this decision. I mean, doctors, we're accustomed to making these decisions. But as relatives, you know, they do it once or twice in their lifetime, and it is

a very hard decision; it's very hard to cope with to see that you have created such a state of grief and regret on the part of someone who gave consent.

A physician working in a small District Stroke Centre also describes how the decision to treat with rt-PA has a profound effect on family members. These family members are not referenced in the discourse promoting the use of this treatment. It is one thing to have a family member die of stroke, he tells me; it is another to have a family member die because of a decision that was made to treat that stroke.

The final step in the process involves actually administering rt-PA for acute stroke. Again, many aspects of this step are taken for granted in textual descriptions that simplify what is actually a complex process. In the following account, a physician working in a community setting describes what happens when the emergency department physicians have initiated a stroke protocol:

> Well, you establish a protocol. But human nature being what it is, the emergency docs, as soon as they make the notification that the patient has a stroke and is a potential rt-PA candidate, then they wash their hands of the case. So you get there to find that the lab work wasn't sent back, that the CT scan is still awaiting, that you know, the blood pressure is sky high and nobody has given them a squirt of anything. So they don't manage the case when they get there. The relatives may not have been spoken to or sought. The patient comes in through the ambulance, so nobody made an effort to find the family so they can provide consent. So those are the types of frustrations that one sees in the real world in the small community hospital. It's a little diluted in a teaching hospital because there is house staff and they deal with all the issues.

This physician has described how the best practice text has been activated[4]—in this instance, a stroke protocol—but he stresses how in the situated practice setting of the community hospital, this gets acted out very differently from what is suggested in the idealized textual account of the written protocol. The protocol is meant to activate a specialized stroke team that doesn't exist. The emergency doctors have assumed the existence of that team and 'washed their hands of the case'. And when the lone specialist does arrive, the entire series of steps outlined in the ideal process has not occurred. The paramedic prompt card, in this instance, has been used to identify the stroke, but this has not been sufficient. The process of ambulance transport has itself hindered the identification of relatives from whom consent can be obtained. The CT scan has not been done because no one was in charge to order it. As the physician concludes, 'It's a little better in a Regional Stroke Centre, but in the community it's difficult'.

## NOTES

1. The NIH Stroke Scale measures nine indicators, seven for language and two for neglect. Because of this, some scientists have argued that the scale favours the detection of left hemisphere strokes, which are those affecting language. In addition, Canada developed its down stroke scale, which is a modified version that is more suitable for administration by nurses.
2. For institutional ethnographies of the work of paramedics, see Corman and Melon (2014); Corman (2017).
3. There are six steps in the application of EBM as it was originally conceived by Sackett and others at McMaster University (Sackett et al., 1997). The patient is examined and a clinical question is constructed. Appropriate resources, such as MedLine are selected, and a literature search is conducted. The selected literature is appraised for its scientific validity. The best evidence, which has been identified from the literature and integrated with clinical expertise and patient preferences, is applied to practice. It is important to note that determining patient preferences and taking them into account is often not well explicated in the literature. Performance is then self-evaluated by the practising physician.
4. On textual activation, see Smith (2005).

## REFERENCES

American Stroke Association. (2003). Guidelines for the early management of patients with ischemic stroke: A scientific statement from the Stroke Council of the American Stroke Association. *Stroke, 34*, 1056–1083.

Corman, M. K. (2017). *Paramedics on and off the streets: Emergency medical services in the age of technological governance*. Toronto, ON: University of Toronto Press.

Corman, M. K., & Melon, K. (2014). What counts? Managing professionals on the front line of emergency services. In A. I. Griffith & D. E. Smith (Eds.), *Under new public management: Institutional ethnographies of changing front-line work* (pp. 149–176). Toronto, ON: University of Toronto Press.

DiLegge, S., Fang, J., Saposnik, G., & Hachinski, V. (2005). The impact of lesion side on acute stroke treatment. *Neurology, 65*, 81–86.

Hand, P. J., Kwan, J., Lindley, R. I., Dennis, M. S., & Wardlaw, J. M. (2006). Distinguishing between stroke and mimic at the bedside: The brain attack study. *Stroke, 37,* 769–775.

Rankin, J. M., & Campbell, M. L. (2006). *Managing to nurse: Inside Canada's health care reform.* Toronto, ON: University of Toronto Press.

Sackett, D. L., Richardson, W. S., Rosenberg, W., & Haynes, R. B. (1997). *Evidence-based Medicine: How to practice and teach EBM.* New York: Churchill Livingstone.

Smith, D. E. (2005). *Institutional ethnography: A sociology for people.* Toronto, ON: AltaMira Press.

Tu, J., & Porter, J. (1999). *Stroke care in Ontario: Hospital survey results.* Toronto, ON: Institute for Clinical Evaluative Sciences.

Wootton, J. (2007). My practice is full and I can't take any new patients. *Canadian Journal of Rural Medicine, 12,* 203–204.

# CHAPTER 6

# A Virtual Success: Evaluation of the Ontario Stroke Strategy

In October 2005, following the release of a report on the evaluation of the Ontario Stroke Strategy (OSS), the Minister of Health published a media release with the headline 'Ontario Stroke Strategy Saving Lives, Improving Access to Life-Saving Treatment'. The evaluation to which the Minister refers was completed during the time period in which I collected my data. In this document, the current Health Minister stated:

> We are ensuring that all Ontarians have access to quality stroke care as soon as possible. We now have put all the pieces in place for a fully functioning regional stroke care system that will ensure that people affected by strokes get the care they need, when and where they need it.

However, some of the accounts provided in this chapter do not support the idea that a 'fully functioning regional stroke care system' has in fact been put in place.

The Minister went on to note that initial evaluation of the Ontario Stroke Strategy by the Stroke Evaluation Advisory Committee (SEAC) indicates that Ontario's stroke care system was already having a positive impact through, among other things, a reduction in 'the time it takes for patients needing life-saving clot-busting drugs to receive treatment ... by ... 35% since 2000'. This would seem an extraordinary success.

What this release *didn't* mention, however, is that these statistics only represented the rates at the participating Regional Stroke Centres (RSCs), which as I have shown are all urban hospitals with access to the best

© The Author(s) 2020
F. Webster, *The Social Organization of Best Practice*,
https://doi.org/10.1007/978-3-030-43165-5_6

technology and resources, including stroke teams and physician specialists. The rate for the use of rt-PA at acute centres continues to be considerably lower. Some of the official literature acknowledges that 'many community and rural hospitals are unable to provide this treatment because of their location or a lack of resources' (Lindsay et al., 2005). Nevertheless, the Ministry of Health continues to document the uptake of thrombolytic therapy (rt-PA) use as part of a core set of indicators for measuring 'optimal' acute care.

Commenting on the evaluation data, a pronouncement was made in a 2004 newsletter of the Canadian Stroke Network (CSN). A high ranking official commented, 'There's no going back ... The strategy will lead to huge improvements in outcomes ... [The] CSN has a registry to gather data and monitor progress in hospitals' (Canadian Stroke Network, 2004). Interestingly, this description suggests that because we have a registry to gather data and 'monitor progress in hospitals', we will necessarily see significant improvements in outcomes. There are several things to note here. First, the focus on gathering data in hospitals means that what we are measuring relates only to the acute episode. But how accurate is this claim? How did it come to be accepted that measuring and monitoring would lead to better outcomes? And by better outcomes, does she mean patient outcomes or economic outcomes?

The assumption that measuring and monitoring will improve stroke care is not backed up by empirical evidence. Anyone who works in health care has heard the statement, 'We cannot manage what we cannot measure'. I have heard it spoken multiple times and have also been at workshops with Peter Drucker, the widely reported author of the quote, in attendance; the quote originated in the business literature, but it was used in 2000 in Ontario to advocate for more and better data in health in order to measure the performance of health care workers and systems. A particular focus of this measurement was on cost. Since that time, health care costs have risen dramatically and are now reported to be consuming more than 50 per cent of many provincial budgets.

If the evaluations of the OSS do not necessarily match the reality 'on the ground' as I have described it in this ethnography, what then could be its purpose? It is in sketching an answer to this question that I am able to render a possible and preliminary link from the Ontario Stroke Strategy to the project of health care reform. Rankin and Campbell's work (2006) explicates the accounting logic that is at the heart of the new public management (NPM) of health care reforms. They draw on the work of

Geoffrey Bowker and Susan Leigh Star to describe the nature of information systems that are currently utilized in the evaluation of health care and that we can see at work in the evaluation of the Stroke Strategy. Rankin and Campbell state:

> We want Canadians to look at so-called successful health care reform. We point out the danger inherent in treating as "truth" the virtual reality that has been generated within and for the purposes of contemporary management practice. This is the knowledge relied on for constructing (or in this case, restructuring) health care. Our analysis offers many instances where objectified textual accounts of people's poor health and suffering and their care and treatment—the stuff of health care—may be adequately represented for the calculation of costs and benefits, *but be deceptive about lives lived in the everyday world* ... As ruling practice, the textual representation supports the work of public policymakers, health planners, and accountants even when their interests are different from health care workers and patients. (Rankin & Campbell, 2006)

The notion of truth as virtual reality describes how evaluation data was used to promote the OSS. The Ontario Stroke Strategy had been developed through data generated through randomized controlled trials (RCTs) and then promoted by epidemiological data generated through provincial evaluations that collect indicators only at specialized Stroke Centres. These numerical and textual accounts produced through the evaluations of the Ontario Stroke Strategy may be deceptive about lives lived in the everyday world.

Nevertheless, providing rt-PA for acute stroke care continues to be an important indicator of a hospital's overall rating. For example, Lindsay et al. (2005) state that 'To achieve "best practice" stroke care across the country, continuous surveillance of the quality of stroke care will become increasingly important' (p. 364). They continue:

> Increasingly, hospitals are being judged on their ability to demonstrate that they are providing "best practice" stroke care. We hope that these indicators will be adopted by hospitals and embedded in routine clinical care as a means of ensuring a minimum standard of practice and to make transparent to front-line clinicians the criteria by which their performance is being judged. Systematic documentation of these indicators on every stroke patient's hospital chart, using standard forms or checklists, should be encouraged. (p. 364)

The discourse of such accounts erases the possibility of exploring if perhaps the evidence, as it was developed in the first place, was not intended to serve the needs of all stroke patients, in all settings, and is perhaps inadequate to do so. I am left reflecting on the words of one community physician who explains it thus:

> The numbers of times I can use [rt-PA] in a small community like this [is small] and every time I use it, it's with some trepidation. So as I say, it's been an advance, but it's not something revolutionary. It's moving stroke care along, but I think we've got just as much out of the recognition that looking after these patients in a detailed and skilful manner is going to accomplish as much as practically any other physician intervention—you know, controlling their blood sugars, controlling their temperature, preventing aspiration, preventing breakdown, urinary tract infections, enrolling them in very early rehabilitation; these things and skilful nursing. All these things that are to me the realization of getting this through the heads of people; looking after stroke has been just as exciting and probably has a greater impact than giving rt-PA to a selected number of patients … If you happen to qualify for rt-PA, along that continuum, so be it. But I don't see it a simple therapy that is going to answer the problems that we have about stroke.

The situated practice for delivering acute stroke care in the community, or at a District Stroke Centre, does not fit the ideal model of the Regional Stroke Centres developed by the Ontario Stroke Strategy. The steps that are easier to implement in an RCT or in an Academic Health Sciences Centre (AHSC) are more difficult to replicate in a community hospital setting. Specifically, it is not easy for patients, their families or onlookers to identify stroke, and in fact it turns out that it is difficult for physicians to identify as well, as we have seen in the previous chapter. Even when paramedics are trained to identify acute stroke, bringing a patient to hospital by ambulance may actually impede the process of delivering care, by separating the patient from their family. In addition, since ambulances do not fall under provincial jurisdiction, emergency personnel may or may not agree to bypass a local hospital to go to a specialized stroke centre, as doing so would tie up many valuable resources. Once at the hospital, a stroke protocol might be initiated even in the absence of a qualified stroke team to then carry out the tasks associated with that protocol. A computed tomography (CT) scanner might not be available, or the appropriate staff with the right expertise might not be available to read the scans. Families or patients may not always be able to absorb information related to acute stroke and thus are unable at times to make an informed decision about the use of rt-PA.

The attempt to standardize the Stroke Strategy treatment across the province does not take these factors into consideration. The medical research of evidence-based medicine (EBM) is specifically designed to eliminate or wash out the effects of situated practices. Yet EBM has to be taken up and put into action by actual people in actual everyday settings of their work. In the ideal setting where rt-PA for acute stroke was developed, a stroke specialist is on call, one who has the support of the emergency department physicians and access to adequate technology as well as radiology staff and specialized nurses. In the situated practice of delivering care, there is a context of physician retention issues, few specialists, lack of technology or staff to interpret CT scans, or both, and few dedicated nursing staff.

If personal experiences do not necessarily shape a physician's treatment decisions, what does? Most of the physicians I interviewed who actively supported the use of rt-PA were neurologists practising in Academic Health Sciences Centres, which were also where the Regional Stroke Centres were located. They had often been involved in the original trials associated with rt-PA. Their excitement about rt-PA for stroke had less to do with the evidence as with the fact that there was now something that could be done at all, as we have seen in the previous chapter. One specialist told me:

> Oh great, for the first time we can use something. I mean, I wanted to jump on the bandwagon of treatment because I grew up in neurology when we didn't have much to offer. So when somebody came along and said, 'Look do you want to do something acutely that can improve outcomes?', I jumped on the bandwagon right away.

I want to draw attention to this statement. The image produced through the medical research discourse is that of the unbiased clinician who appraises the scientific evidence and then decides whether or not to use it in any particular instance. What was driving this specialist, who deals exclusively with acute stroke, was the fact that 'for the first time we can use something'. He 'jumps on the bandwagon right away'. He has reasons, good ones, beyond the science base to implement this new treatment. This type of institutional factor related to medical decision-making is rarely described in the knowledge translation (KT) discourse.

Early in my analysis I created a map (see Fig. 6.1) showing the relationships between the Regional and District Stroke Centres, the community physicians and the OSS. The map shows how in the model of the OSS, the specialist's working knowledge has been central to the development of the OSS and the specialist occupies the position of initiator or innovator. *The specialist is also the person who has the connection with the medical research discourse through participation in RCTs.* Not surprisingly, in my study the specialists working at Regional (and sometimes District) Stroke Centres were most likely to be involved in producing the evidence for acute stroke. They were also most likely to promote its use. In addition to being developed in urban, specialized settings, and perhaps because of this, rt-PA is most useful within those settings. In the community setting, access to such treatment varies with several central features of organization, as I have outlined previously in this book.

Despite the relative absence of debate amongst the physicians I spoke with regarding the scientific evidence for rt-PA, it is worth noting that its acceptance as best practice care did not come about readily. Following the National Institute of Neurological Disorders and Stroke (NINDS) Trial in August 2000, the American Heart Association (AHA) upgraded its

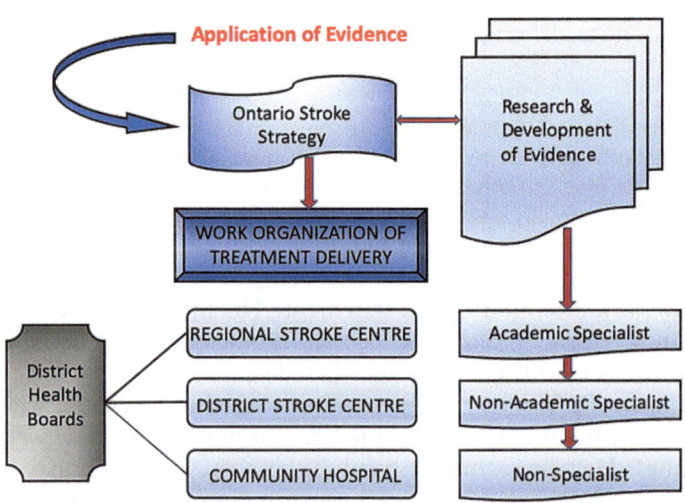

**Fig. 6.1** Organizational structure informing physician decision-making

recommendation of rt-PA for acute stroke from an optional class to a Class 1 definitely recommended (Lenzer, 2002). Some felt that this recommendation came despite continued concerns about the safety and efficacy of the treatment. I will summarize these concerns here. First, the recommendation by the American Heart Association was based on one trial. Unlike the NINDS Trial results, most other randomized controlled trials (RCTs) have shown that thrombolysis (the dissolution of dangerous blood clots) *increases* mortality in acute ischemic stroke. In addition, many more patients in the treatment arm had mild stroke scores at baseline, while more in the placebo arm had worse scores. Therefore, at least some percentage of those patients in the treatment arm had symptoms that would have resolved themselves without any intervention. In addition, the external validity of this particular trial has been questioned, since the proportion of patients enrolled in the 0–90-minute group was artificially increased through study design criteria. Chance alone could explain the benefit shown in this single study.

Because many physicians did question the scientific validity of evidence produced through a single study, the European Medicines Evaluation Agency (EMEA) called for another RCT to establish its efficacy. In response to this challenge of the scientific evidence, various clinical and observational studies were undertaken to see if real-life experiences of delivering rt-PA for acute stroke would mirror those of the NINDS Trial. For instance, one study followed patients treated with rt-PA from December 1, 1998, to February 1, 2000, at a Regional Stroke Centre in Ontario (Silver et al., 2001). The NINDS criteria were followed, except for one major exception. Patients with less severe stroke were not included. Compared to the NINDS Trial, more patients were treated after 90 minutes and also tended to be older, factors associated with poorer outcomes. Despite this, the results of the NINDS Trial were matched and even excelled. The authors conclude that 'imaging exclusion criteria may optimize the benefits of rt-PA'. Proponents of the use of rt-PA for acute stroke now marshalled this additional—although less robust—evidence (according to EBM standards) to support their advocacy for its use.

However, this 'real-life study' was still conducted at a Regional Stroke Centre, in turn housed at an Academic Health Sciences Centre. The improvement in results was related to better imaging achieved through CT scans that were expertly read by specialized radiologists. And efficacy in expert hands is not the same as clinical effectiveness in usual clinical practice. Through the OSS, this intervention was standardized as best practice and implemented in settings very different from that where it was originally designed.

## DEBATES ABOUT WHO SHOULD PROVIDE RT-PA

One of the key questions that arose in relation to this treatment was that of who should deliver the therapy. The emergency stroke patient arrives at the emergency department and will be assessed by an emergency physician, who in the community setting is typically also a family physician. Yet the Canadian Association of Emergency Room Physicians (CAEP) issued a position statement in January 2001 that questioned the scientific evidence for the determination of stroke. They stated that 'until it is clear that the benefits of this therapy outweigh the risks, thrombolytic therapy for acute stroke should be restricted to use within formal research protocols or in monitored practice protocols that adhere to the NINDS eligibility criteria' (Canadian Association of Emergency Physicians, 2001, p. 11). They recommended limiting the role of the emergency physician to identifying stroke and initiating CT scans but urged that 'only physicians with demonstrated expertise in neuroradiology should interpret head CT scans used to determine whether to administer thrombolytic agents to stroke patients. Neurologists should be directly involved prior to the thrombolytic administration' (p. 8). In these statements, one can see emerging the different professional standpoints informing the experience of physicians.

The CAEP position statement led to many arguments taking place in medical journals and at conferences. In these exchanges, the discourse of EBM was drawn upon to debate the evidence for and against the use of rt-PA for acute stroke. For example, in the journal *Stroke*, the editors argued that awareness of the risks and benefits of rt-PA was insufficient 'regardless of specialty' and further argued that 'an unjustified fear' of rt-PA side effects might limit a patient's access to this treatment (Katzan, Sila, & Furlan, 2001). In this discourse, then, the issue of patient access becomes the discursive moral centre of the argument for rt-PA and notions about individual physicians' feelings or attitudes are to blame for their 'insufficient' practice.

Indeed, most urban specialists I interviewed attributed the variation in use of rt-PA for stroke in community settings to irrational fear on the part of the community physicians. They tended to make this judgement even when it contradicted their experience. As one specialist stated, 'I don't know of any [doctors] personally that don't give it, but I know from the literature that people are afraid of it'. 'Knowing from the literature' is a phrase that provides an example of how the discourse produced through texts is taken up as reality. As Rankin and Campbell (2006) have noted in their study of the impact of Canada's health care reform on nursing practice, knowledge produced through statistics represents a virtual reality that overrides the professional's own experiences (p. 55). In this instance, the specialist describes how he 'knows from the literature' that others are 'afraid of rt-PA' for their patients. This specialist then acknowledges that the fearful physicians he is describing 'might not have neurosurgical backup in their local hospitals'. Therefore, it would seem, their fear is valid. Fear of haemorrhage is different from the knowledge that one does not have neurosurgical backup in their local hospitals. The one is a psychological fear of possible negative outcomes, while the other is recognition of lack of structural resources.

Several physicians expressed their belief that the fear of delivering rt-PA reflects a difference in personality between emergency room physicians and stroke specialists. In the following account, a specialist is emphatic that the fear must be disregarded and also stresses that evidence from the literature ('when case studies are fully published') will reduce that fear. Thus, the solution to fear will be information. He says:

> Yea, I think we've got to get over this fear. Emergency physicians have been pretty reluctant about this whole thing because they don't want to be landed with it. And this is just the situation that has been done for cardiology; well, why not for neurology—but I think they're scared. The difference is that the brain bleeds and the heart doesn't, basically, and so therefore they're nervous, and obviously there are more parameters we have to evaluate in a stroke case as compared to a cardiac case. I think I can understand their reluctance, but when the case studies are fully published and emphasized, our Canadian study, I think that will help also to improve that [feeling of nervousness], as far as this perception goes with the emergency physicians.

In a survey published in 2005, 1105 emergency physicians in the United States indicated that they were unlikely to give stroke patients rt-PA, even in an ideal setting, mostly because of their concerns of causing brain bleeding (Brown, Barsan, Lisabeth, Gallery, & Morgenstern, 2005). But the majority of doctors from this study also said that if they had appropriate backup from neurologists and the right personnel to help them diagnose and treat appropriate patients, they would give rt-PA. Obviously, having appropriate personnel and backup aren't considered part of the ideal setting according to this survey. Another specialist told me:

> I think reluctance on the part of the emergency doctors is that they don't want to be made responsible for the interpretation of CT scans ... so unless you make available to them real-time interpretation of CT scans—wouldn't it be nice if we had a test, a component for the brain that would let them know that this is in fact what's happening.

Efforts have been made for specialists in Regional Centres to provide real-time interpretation of CT scans through telestroke. Telestroke is designed to allow specialists working in Regional Stroke Centres to read CT scans taken in other sites and thus increase the use of rt-PA in remote or semi-rural areas. But of course the introduction of this approach imposes a new set of difficulties. As Italian sociologist Nicolini (2005) observes, the tendency of technology in medicine is to modify the existing coordination of health care services 'in the direction of existing centres of power, both professional and economical' (p. 2756). In the case of stroke, an argument can be made that interventions such as rt-PA for acute stroke clearly modify the existing or previous coordination in favour of special-ized centres that have access to the technology and human resources to carry out best evidence therapies. It also privileges which types of patients can receive the best standard care. As one study found (You, Venkatesh, & Laupacis, 2009), the recent investment in Ontario in magnetic resonance imaging (MRI) scanning doubled the utilization of these machines over five years. However, 'utilization increased disproportionately for those liv-ing in the richest neighbourhoods' (You et al., 2009, p. 23). They also conclude that it is not clear if more access to MRI will result in better outcomes.

## THE PATIENT'S BODY AS A SITE FOR CONDUCTING RESEARCH

Some EBM research has focused on doctor–patient communication (Ford, Schofield, & Hope, 2003; Haynes, Devereaux, & Guyatt, 2002), although critical scholars have argued that the technologies of EBM do not ade-quately take into account patient preferences (Mykhalovskiy, 2003). Currently, the notion of shared decision-making is coming into use as a model for understanding and improving the role of the patient in clinical decision-making (Légaré et al., 2008). Yet the extent to which can patients engage meaningfully in conversations about their medical care is not well understood.

Instead, research into why patients do not participate in research is often explored from the perspective of learning how to better seek their participation in clinical trials (Whitstock, 2003). For example, one qualitative study interviewed patients who were recruited to an epilepsy treatment trial with the explicit goal of learning how to train future trial recruiters (Canvin & Jacoby, 2006). The researchers labelled patients who did not participate in research as having weak altruism. The moral imperative that faces physicians to become researchers also plays a role in how patients are constructed as altruistic in their willingness to contribute to the development of scientific knowledge; their study found that some patients participate in research trials as a way to achieve clinical treatment. This can be seen in the following account of a patient named William[1] at a stroke clinic. He tells me:

> I could have used some more information about foods; I could have got it had I thought to ask; but at the time I didn't. I was told the dos, but I wasn't told the don'ts. Maybe that wasn't necessary, and I wasn't told that, and I have wondered about that. I was able to straighten that out this morning in the interview I had [i.e., with a specialist]. Yes, that was the real purpose [to participate in research]. I wasn't supposed to see [doctor name], I was to see his nurse who is coordinating this study. But I brought up a series of questions, so I ended up seeing the doctor as well, although it wasn't intended [for me to do that].

William understands that the 'real purpose' of his visit was as a research subject. Through his participation, he is able to access a physician so as to be able to ask more questions related to his concerns around food and symptoms. Patients at community hospitals, or who are patients with physicians who do not run studies, would not have this type of access. I ask William what his next steps will be in terms of his medical care; again, we see how his role as a study participant is intricately interwoven with his status as a patient receiving care. William describes what will happen next in his care:

> Well, the first step is this heart scan that I'm going to have probably within the next couple of weeks. And then I'm involved in this study—[it is] just starting, so I don't really know exactly in detail what's going to happen, but

it does involve medication, 50 per cent of which is a placebo, and I'll never know which one I'm on. And then I'll be contacted every couple of weeks by telephone, and also I'll have the conferences, maybe three to four times a year, about that [i.e., kind of timing]. And I think as far as I'm aware right now, that's about it.

The practice of evidence-based medicine is based on clinical trials that take place in ideal conditions. The medical research of EBM is specifically designed to eliminate or wash out the effects of what I have referred to as situated practices. The process for developing and testing the evidence for rt-PA was not as simple or as obvious as it would appear on the surface. Evidence was achieved through one randomized controlled trial in which only ideal patients were selected for participation and at sites in which a high degree of technological expertise was available. Not everyone agreed that the evidence for rt-PA warranted its uptake by such organizations as the American Heart Association.

The development of research through clinical trials has important consequences for those patients who participate and for those who do not, as well as for nurses and other hospital staff. Little is known about the patient's experiences of participating in clinical trials. It is an important and often invisible part of the coordination of the production of knowledge for the evidence base as well as for delivery of care. Studies exploring the patient's standpoint often explicitly conduct their analysis with a view to increase patient participation in research. Patients who do not consent to participate are viewed as having weak altruism. According to my interviews, research also can deleteriously affect the work of nursing when the patient's participation in research directly contradicts how nurses have been asked to care for their patients. Finally, when access to additional care is provided to patients through their participation in research, how can we meaningfully speak of providing equitable access to those patients who do not live close to teaching hospitals?

## NOTE

1. Pseudonyms were used to protect the identity of all participants.

# References

Brown, D. L., Barsan, W. G., Lisabeth, L. D., Gallery, M. E., & Morgenstern, L. B. (2005). Survey of emergency physicians about recombinant tissue plasminogen activator for acute ischemic stroke. *Annals of Emergency Medicine, 46*, 56–60.

Canadian Association of Emergency Physicians (CAEP), & Committee on Thrombolytic Therapy for Acute Ischemic Stroke. (2001). Position statement: Thrombolytic therapy for acute ischemic stroke. *Canadian Journal of Emergency Medicine, 3*, 8–12.

Canadian Stroke Network. (2004). *Canadian Stroke Network Newsletter, 4,* 2, 1–3.

Canvin, K., & Jacoby, A. (2006). Duty, desire or indifference? A qualitative study of patient decisions about recruitment to an epilepsy treatment trial. *Trials Journal, 7,* 32.

Ford, S., Schofield, T., & Hope, T. (2003). What are the ingredients for a successful evidence-based patient choice consultation? A qualitative study. *Social Science & Medicine, 56,* 589–602.

Haynes, R. B., Devereaux, P. J., & Guyatt, G. H. (2002). Physicians' and patients' choices in evidence based practice. *British Medical Journal, 324,* 1350. https://doi.org/10.1186/1745-6215-7-32

Katzan, I. L., Sila, C., & Furlan, A. J. (2001). Community use of intravenous tissue plasminogen activator for acute stroke: Results of the brain matters stroke management survey. *Stroke, 32,* 861–864.

Légaré, F., Elwyn, G., Fishbein, M., Fremont, P., Frosch, D., Kenny, D. A., et al. (2008). Translating shared decision-making into health care clinical practices: Proof of concepts. *Implementation Science, 3,* 2. https://doi.org/10.1186/1748-5908-3-2

Lenzer, J. (2002). Alteplase for stroke: Money and optimistic claims buttress the brain attack campaign. *British Medical Journal, 324,* 723–729.

Lindsay, M. P., Kapral, M. K., Gladstone, D., Holloway, R., Tu, J. V., Laupacis, A., et al. (2005). The Canadian Stroke Quality of Care Study: Establishing indicators for optimal acute stroke care. *Canadian Medical Association Journal, 172,* 363–365.

Mykhalovskiy, E. (2003). Evidence-based medicine: Ambivalent reading and the clinical recontextualization of science. *Health: An Interdisciplinary Journal for the Social Study of Health, Illness and Medicine, 7,* 331–352.

Nicolini, D. (2005). The work to make telemedicine work: A social and articulate view. *Social Science & Medicine, 62,* 2754–2767.

Rankin, J. M., & Campbell, M. L. (2006). *Managing to nurse: Inside Canada's health care reform.* Toronto, ON: University of Toronto Press.

Silver, B., Demaerschalk, B., Merino, J. G., Wong, E., Tamayo, A., Devasenapathy, A., et al. (2001). Improved outcomes in stroke thrombolysis with pre-specified imaging criteria. *Canadian Journal of Neurological Sciences, 28*, 113–119.

Whitstock, M. T. (2003). Seeking evidence from medical research consumers as part of the medical research process could improve the uptake of research evidence. *Journal of Evaluation in Clinical Practice, 9*, 213–224.

You, J. J., Venkatesh, V., & Laupacis, A. (2009). Better access to outpatient magnetic resonance imaging in Ontario: But for whom? *Open Medicine, 3*(1), 22–25.

# CHAPTER 7

# Conclusion

In October 2006, the Heart and Stroke Foundation of Ontario launched a new advertising campaign heralding its involvement in the use of rt-PA for acute stroke; such advertising continues to this day. This emphasized, once again, the acute care episode and the notion of an almost magical cure. The idea of preventing stroke, or of coordinating and improving services across the continuum of care, including the provision of rehabilitation, becomes lost from view. In the television advertisement, a flower droops while a narrator speaks of the devastating effects of stroke. Then, thrombolytic therapy (rt-PA) is described, and the flower is shown returning to its original glory, intact and blooming. This is the Lazarus Effect and it is compelling.

However, fewer than 10 per cent of patients are ever eligible for this treatment, and outside of urban centres, this number is far lower. And of those 10 per cent who are eligible, far less will experience the Lazarus Effect. In the original National Institute of Neurological Disorders and Stroke (NINDS) Trial, the benefit from rt-PA was seen at three months. As one specialist commented to me,

> I don't expect Lazarus to rise from the dead, and I caution people on the risks and benefits of it and tell them that in the study it was apparent at the 90-day mark [that] there was a difference between treatment with placebo. I have not been blessed with patents that jump off the emergency room table thanking me for giving them rt-PA.

© The Author(s) 2020
F. Webster, *The Social Organization of Best Practice*,
https://doi.org/10.1007/978-3-030-43165-5_7

The physicians with whom I worked and who I interviewed did not work in isolation. Their access to resources, both human and technological, seemed to shape their decision-making more profoundly than their appraisal of the evidence for rt-PA for acute stroke. It was not, in other words, that the evidence for rt-PA for acute stroke was questioned as being scientifically sound. It was that rt-PA for acute stroke did not suit the local context in which they practised medicine.

Throughout this book, and using the example of rt-PA for acute stroke, I have argued against the concept of the physician problem as an explanatory model for why best practice medicine is not more widely practised. I have argued that the Ontario Stroke Strategy (OSS) was organized around acute care services from the outset, as this is where randomized controlled trials (RCTs) were conducted and would produce the 'gold standard evidence' of care. It is rare that RCTs can be conducted for health promotion or primary prevention interventions, for many complex reasons (Colditz & Taylor, 2010). Thus, these sectors are considered less evidence-based and as a result become unlikely to garner the type of resources necessary to ensure success. Indeed these sectors of the care continuum were not evaluated as indicators were only collected from the acute care settings of Regional Stroke Centres (RSCs).

Some have argued that the evidence-based discourse is an example of 'microfascism' within the contemporary scientific arena (Holmes, Murray, Perron, & Rail, 2006). Holmes and his team draw attention to how the evidence-based health sciences represent a Foucauldian 'regime of truth' wherein only one form of truth, in this case the one produced through the RCT, is allowed as fact, thus dismissing 98 per cent of all research. As I have noted, systematic reviews begin with a broad search of the research literature, which identifies hundreds or thousands of articles on a topic. Next, all of those articles not based on rigorously designed RCTs or not reported properly are excluded. The authors then typically review and consider the results from the remaining studies, which is typically a small proportion (e.g., 10–50 per cent) of the research articles identified in the search. Yet all the excluded articles were published in peer-reviewed journals and were therefore deemed to be valid research information by academic peer reviewers. Holmes and his co-authors also point out how the current literature ignores the relational aspects of knowledge and dismisses the role of values in health care. For them, 'the clinician can often be considered such an institutional subject who is presumed both to know the truth of disease and to have the moral and intellectual authority to prescribe treatment' (Holmes et al., 2006, p. 183).

My study explored the actual setting in which physicians provided care and made decisions about whether or not to treat a patient with rt-PA. In undertaking this study, I soon discovered that the Academic Health Sciences Centres (AHSCs) were also the sites for producing evidence, as nurses and physicians I interviewed participated in clinical trials. In this study, those most likely to be involved in the production of knowledge were also those most likely to promote the new therapies produced through meta-analyses or RCTs. This insight goes beyond dichotomous arguments for and against the uses of evidence and beyond abstract theories about how to disseminate evidence to physicians or encouraging them to change. Rather, it draws attention to what physicians actually do in the everyday worlds of delivering care and making decisions. What emerged consistently from the accounts I gathered is that stroke care was coordinated in ways that often overlooked the everyday conditions under which the individual physician was working. And this coordination masked particular institutional interests that determined the delivery of this acute treatment rather than individual decision-making.

Originally, the types of medical practice that were the focus of evidence-based medicine (EBM) efforts were widely considered by most experts as clearly beneficial and quite straightforward. A commonly cited example is that of the use of Vitamin C to prevent scurvy (Timmermans & Berg, 2003). A more recent example would be hand hygiene in hospitals, for example, which remains an area of concern and results in a high percentage of unnecessary infections every year in Canadian hospitals (Vermeil et al., 2019); it would seem self-evident that getting physicians to use the best practice hand-washing techniques is important. Critical scholars in other fields have noted how such self-evident explanations may act as a barrier to empirical study of how work is organized. For example, in discussing the ideological frame of multiculturalism, Ng observes that 'commonsensical' explanations work to replace any need to study what is actually going on (Ng, 1995). In much the same way, it has become increasingly accepted that translating knowledge into clinical care and ensuring uptake will improve patient care and patient outcomes. This seems so 'commonsensical' that there is no need to study what is actually going on.

When we uncritically accept that the evidence produced through meta-analyses of RCTs is 'best', we inadvertently erase the work processes through which that knowledge was produced. This allows for strong moral pronouncements by knowledge translation (KT) specialists against physicians who do not make use of 'best' evidence in their work. The terms best practice and best evidence as used in clinical guidelines call up the ethical principle of doing no harm that forms the background of physician practice. It implies that the only alternative to best care would be less good care.

The knowledge exists that there are systemic and structural reasons for the failure of rt-PA to be taken up widely. In essence, the entire OSS is designed to restructure the delivery of health care services in order to facilitate the uptake of this treatment without adding additional resources. The OSS However, established and attempted to standardize an ideal model of care that did not account for the various contextual settings in which the everyday work of clinical care was provided. Even when the local context is recognized, it often becomes a problem to be solved, rather than being considered a reflection of broader issues related to the organization of health care services. Lambert (2005) has noted what she terms the 'assimilationist nature' of EBM. She states:

> My review of the literature suggests that criticism has characteristically been countered not by rejection, contestation, or entrenchment, but by incorporation. This assimilationist response is fairly characteristic of the way in which biomedicine, as an institutionally dominant system, has dealt in many country contexts with other (traditional, indigenous and alternative) medical traditions. (p. 4)

In a similar manner, and since the time that I undertook my study, the OSS has responded to some of the problems in implementation I have described by attempting to incorporate solutions to emerging problems without shifting the organizing framework that prioritizes one set of interests over another. A key example is the establishment of telestroke. As noted in this book, telestroke is designed to allow specialists working in Regional Stroke Centres to read computed tomography (CT) scans taken in other sites and thus increase the use of rt-PA in remote or semi-rural areas. But it cannot be provided 24/7 and puts a significant burden on the specialists at those very Regional Stroke Centres. It also continues to place effort and resources at the acute level of care rather than that of prevention. Future studies will hopefully discover how telestroke and other technological strategies designed to address gaps that arise across the continuum are affecting the everyday work performed by care providers at Regional and District Stroke Centres, as well as at community hospitals.

I originally set out wanting to know what was 'wrong' with those physicians who were choosing not to deliver rt-PA for acute stroke. Through my study, I discovered a disjuncture between the best practice treatments developed through clinical trials and promoted through texts, such as the Blue Book, and the actualities of their translation into practice. Smith (2005) wrote:

> Institutional Ethnography is essentially a work of inquiry and discovery; it must move beyond what the ethnographer already knows or thinks she or he knows, and the ethnographer must be prepared for and open to finding out that matters are not as he or she may have envisaged them. (p. 207)

Through finding out what physicians actually do in their work, including their relationships with others in the health care system, I was able to discover forms of coordination—in particular those with the Ontario Stroke Strategy—that were largely invisible in accounts of scientific evidence and physician decision-making. The physicians I spoke with did not decide to deliver rt-PA according to their appraisal of the evidence. Few physicians in any location, urban teaching centre or hospital, questioned the validity of the original NINDS Trial for rt-PA. They also did they not report any reliance on their personal experiences of delivering this treatment.

What did emerge consistently from the accounts is that the coordination of stroke care through the OSS was designed without taking into consideration the everyday conditions under which the individual physician was working. And this coordination is what seemed to determine the successful delivery of this acute treatment for stroke. This in and of itself is a relatively simple point and has been documented elsewhere. For example, one Canadian study examined community factors, hospital characteristics and inter-regional outcome variations following acute myocardial infarction (heart attack) in Canada (Alter, Austin, & Tu, 2004). Their research also supported the idea that 'supply factors affect physician decision-making processes' (p. 254). That is to say, physicians with access to technology and advanced treatments will be more likely to use them. Again, this would seem a self-evident point in some respects. What remains unexamined is how health care is coordinated so that, despite clinicians' emphasis on the need for prevention, the majority of funds are directed towards acute care and post-event pharmaceutical therapies.

Within Canada, the push to develop standards of care based on best evidence health care continues through such organizations as the Canadian Institutes for Health Research (CIHR). CIHR will not fund research studies that do not have a knowledge translation component. The OSS continued to channel $30 million per year into the organization of stroke care services that are organized primarily around the delivery of acute services, despite the claim to improve equitable access across the continuum of care. The Canadian Stroke Network, 2000–2014 was established, based on the Ontario model, with funding from the Canadian Stroke Network as well as the provinces. Yet the analysis of data collected from the Regional Stroke Centres by the Registry of the Canadian Stroke Network (RCSN) concluded that 'we do not yet have data on long-term stroke outcomes such as mortality and functional status, so we cannot evaluate the association between the processes of stroke care and stroke outcomes' (Kapral et al., 2004, p. 1760). That is to say, the data that has been collected cannot show whether or not standards for stroke care, such as rt-PA, have been implemented. There is also *no known connection* between meeting the standards of care and improving patient outcomes following stroke. Given the emphasis on best practice care that is so dominant within the EBM discourse, this is an extraordinary admission.

The best practice stroke care on which hospitals should be judged is not linked to patient outcomes; such practice may or may not improve or save a patient's life. And yet the assertion is made that systematic documentation of these indicators—using standardized forms or checklists—should be encouraged. The textual basis of the OSS comes full circle. The evidence that produced rt-PA for acute stroke as a best practice was developed through the specific technologies of EBM; that evidence then became the basis for the Ontario Stroke System, which produced the ideal model for care delivery that was arguably focused on acute care. Evaluation of the OSS then evaluated specifically those indicators that reflected both acute care and the realities of the specialized Regional Stroke Centres. On this basis, the model was deemed successful.

Knowledge translation strategies continue to be developed to target individual physicians. Far from being a lone practitioner making decisions autonomously, I found that the physicians I spoke with were involved with an entire network of others in their everyday work. The decisions that they made relied upon the presence of many others active in the care delivery situation, including technicians, radiologists, nurses, paramedics, pharmaceutical staff and of course patients and their families. They were not out of date or old; neither were they ignorant of best practice evidence, nor did they resist using it.

Another tendency in the KT discourse has been towards involving end users in the production of research. This sounds harmless enough and in fact echoes the spirit of participant research in some ways. It would also seem to hold the answer to the problem of local context; that is, involving those who are likely to deliver care in the development of research. Despite theoretical acceptance of this principle, it doesn't appear to be happening in practice. Who are these end users, how are they identified and what role do they play in shaping the direction of research? We need to pay attention to this question rather than accept uncritically that their involvement in research will necessarily lead to better patient care.

Finally, I want to clarify that through this analysis, I am not arguing against the validity of scientific knowledge or biomedical research or suggesting that the neurologists involved in RCTs were in some way uncaring or self-interested. I have attempted instead to render visible how care has been coordinated so that various standpoints, such as that of the stroke specialist, are taken up in the creation of ideal models—such as that outlined in the evidence-based Blue Book—and then transferred to local settings.

Evidence-based medicine can be conceived of as a discourse that informs how the relationship between scientific knowledge and medical practice is thought to be ideally coordinated. In this discourse, delays in bringing basic science advances into clinical practice are said to cause patients untold harm every year. Writing an editorial in a leading medical journal, Rosenberg (2003) pronounced that 'The American people need to know that the current system for bringing promising biomedical research to the bedside is operating at an obsolete level of efficiency, causing great delay, and consequently resulting in the loss of many lives' (p. 1306). His comment could as well have been written today. The idea that promising biomedical research can indeed be quickly brought to the bedside in order to save lives is not backed up by scientific or empirical evidence to this day. But this argument does reveal very clearly some of the competition for resources within health care that takes place in relation to evidence-based medicine. It is also representative of how science is generally constructed within this literature. It is objective and neutral and can be readily used for the public good. Any delays in its use are unethical. So we are led to believe.

For those patients who are eligible, thrombolytic therapy can be life-saving and can dramatically improve their quality of life post-stroke. The focus on acute therapies for stroke has also created an opportunity to improve how stroke patients are cared for post-stroke through the development of an organized system, the Ontario Stroke Strategy. However, the issue is not as simply defined as determining if one particular therapy is useful or not for some patients. There is increasing emphasis for physicians and patients to become involved in the production of new scientific and acute-based knowledge, regardless of how these new treatments may or may not be practical to implement across various settings. This emphasis on new knowledge also erases the need to increase resources and expand other forms of knowledge in relation to areas such as prevention and rehabilitation. This affects both their everyday working lives and the everyday working lives of nurses and other health care practitioners. And as I have only touched on here, it may also significantly affect patients whose bodies become the site of knowledge production.

The guiding aim of the OSS has been to provide equitable access to care across the care continuum. My work has suggested that the continuum is largely ideological and may not exist in actual practice situations. In institutional ethnography (IE),

> Ideological discourses are generalized and generalizing discourses, operating at a metalevel to control other discourses, including institutional discourses … Institutional discourses select those aspects of what people do that are accountable within it, subsuming actualities [i.e., people's work as coordinated by texts] as integral to the production of the institution. (Smith, 2005, pp. 224–225)

As Campbell and Manicom point out, ideology is something that is done in practice (1995, p. xi); it is something accomplished in everyday activity as coordinated by ruling texts such as the Blue Book. It is people in their activity who produce evidence-based medicine. The OSS has been based on the premise that good scientific evidence exists for the notion that 'strokes can be prevented and acute care and rehabilitation appreciably enhanced' (Joint Stroke Strategy Working Group, 2000, p. 2). Yet only the acute care point of care has been emphasized and resourced; this has affected the extent to which prevention and rehabilitation have been 'enhanced'. The ideological discourse can be seen at work here, framing how care is provided (or not).

In a certain sense, my study highlights what has been defined in more recent years as the problem of 'context' in implementing best practice care. However, this is a rather simple conceptualization of a complex problem that does not identify differing institutional priorities or interests, and obfuscates trans-local coordination. It suggests that neutral actors simply practice differently depending on their contexts. The conduct of practice in medicine continues to focus on specific guidelines for practical intervention rather than an examination of the structural conditions and institutional interests that largely influence what becomes identified as best practice.

This study can be thought of as another piece of the puzzle of how health care is coordinated using the approach of institutional ethnography. Building on the work of a small but growing group of IE researchers doing work in the area of health care, I set out to study the concrete forms of coordination that informed physician use of acute stroke therapies. Throughout my study I drew upon their various contributions to understanding how ruling relations are achieved in health care and how this both is created by and influences the actions of real people working in particular settings. For example, I draw upon Rankin and Campbell's study of nursing work in achieving health care reform and in particular take up their notion of how virtual realities are created by the new information technologies, such as administrative databases (Rankin & Campbell, 2006). The notion of virtual realities is relevant to my study in which physician and hospital performance related to acute stroke is measured and evaluated through information collected through the Canadian Stroke Registry. These textual realities are then used to further legitimize and privilege the use of a particular pharmaceutical intervention.

The evidence base, I would suggest, does not need to be dismissed but perhaps as, anthropologist Helen Lambert (2005) points out, 'negotiated and broadened' (p. 2). Until knowledge translation strategies are developed that take into account the institutional interests that inform how medical care is delivered, and the relational aspects of decision-making are acknowledged, it is unlikely that efforts to eliminate variation in practice will be successful. In addition, the role of industry will remain less visible despite their strong role in shaping what is considered best practice through the funding of trials that favour pharmaceutical interventions or medical devices. Through this lens, variation in practice and local context become more than just problems to be solved. They may in fact highlight that the narrow band of strategies for which we have evidence supports interests that organize not just individual physician practice but also priorities at the institutional level of hospitals, governments and health charities. Such interests are erased by the discursive claims to improve care 'across the continuum'.

The number of intervention studies has increased dramatically since the time of this ethnography and the commitment to develop and advance best practice evidence from systematic reviews of RCTs has if anything strengthened. Tremendous effort and extensive funding are directed towards developing innovative strategies to translate, transfer and improve the uptake of research findings in clinical and policy settings. More contemporary terms have entered the lexicon of a field that is now known as Implementation Science, terms such as spread, innovation and patient-centred care. And yet from my vantage point there is still not a corresponding shift in understanding whose knowledge is privileged through best practice care and what institutional priorities are leading the science which we all clamour to bring into practice. Until the politics underlying the social production of knowledge in EBM are addressed and institutional interests laid bare, urgent health care issues such as health disparities and the need for a robust public health system—issues that are not amenable to trials of pharmaceutical interventions—will continue to be underfunded and unresolved. The promise of 'equitable access to care across the continuum' will remain only an unrealized dream not just for stroke care but in relation to most health conditions.

## References

Alter, D. A., Austin, P., & Tu, J. (2004). Community factors, hospital characteristics and inter-regional outcome variations following acute myocardial infarction in Canada. *Canadian Journal of Cardiology, 21*(3), 247–255.

Campbell, M., & Manicom, A. (1995). Foreword. In M. Campbell & A. Manicom (Eds.), *Knowledge, experience, and ruling relations: Studies in the social organization of knowledge* (pp. ix–xv). Toronto, ON: University of Toronto Press.

Colditz, G. A., & Taylor, P. R. (2010). Prevention trials: Their place in how we understand the value of prevention strategies. *Annual Review of Public Health, 31*, 105–120. https://doi.org/10.1146/annurev.publhealth.121208.131051

Holmes, D., Murray, S. J., Perron, A., & Rail, G. (2006, September 4). Deconstructing the evidence-based discourse in health sciences: Truth, power and fascism. *International Journal of Evidence-based Healthcare, 4*(3), 180–186. https://doi.org/10.1111/j.1479-6988.2006.00041.x

Joint Stroke Strategy Working Group. (2000). *Towards an integrated stroke strategy for Ontario*. Toronto, ON: Ministry of Health and Long-Term Care.

Kapral, M. K., Laupacis, A., Phillips, S. J., Silver, F. L., Hill, M. D., Fang, J., et al. (2004). Stroke care delivery in institutions participating in the Registry of the Canadian Stroke Network. *Stroke, 35*, 1756–1762.

Lambert, H. (2005). Accounting for EBM: Notions of evidence in medicine. *Social Science & Medicine, 62*, 2633–2645.

Ng, R. (1995). Multiculturalism as ideology: A textual analysis. In M. Campbell & A. Manicom (Eds.), *Knowledge, experience, and ruling relations* (pp. 35–48). Toronto, ON: University of Toronto Press.

Rankin, J. M., & Campbell, M. L. (2006). *Managing to nurse: Inside Canada's health care reform*. Toronto, ON: University of Toronto Press.

Rosenberg, R. N. (2003). Translating biomedical research to the bedside. *Journal of the American Medical Association, 289*, 1305–1306.

Smith, D. E. (2005). *Institutional ethnography: A sociology for people*. Toronto, ON: AltaMira.

Timmermans, S., & Berg, M. (2003). *The gold standard: The challenge of evidence-based medicine and standardization in health care*. Philadelphia: Temple University Press.

Vermeil, T., Peters, A., Kilpatrick, C., Pires, D., Allegranzi, B., & Pittet, D. (2019). Hand hygiene in hospitals: Anatomy of a revolution. *Journal of Hospital Infection, 101*(4), 383–392.

# Appendix A: Ministry of Health and Long-Term Care (MOHLTC)—Ontario Stroke Strategy (OSS)

## Service Guidelines: District Stroke Centres (DSC)

### Section A

**DSC Role**
- The DSC is accountable, in conjunction with their Regional Stroke Centre (RSC), to provide leadership, development, implementation and integration of stroke care throughout their district and across all points in the spectrum of stroke care (promotion, primary and secondary prevention, acute care, rehabilitation and home care).
- The DSC will assist community hospitals in their district to localize and implement stroke protocols and stroke teams.
- The DSC coordinates and assists the community-based agencies responsible for health promotion and stroke prevention in building inter-organizational relationships throughout their respective catchment areas and across the spectrum of stroke care.
- The DSC is committed to participating in ongoing education/training in stroke care within their region and providing an integrated stroke service based on best practices.

© The Author(s) 2020
F. Webster, *The Social Organization of Best Practice*,
https://doi.org/10.1007/978-3-030-43165-5

**Accountability**

- In partnership with the Regional Stroke Steering Committees (RSSC) and the RSCs the DSCs are accountable for the leadership, development, implementation and coordination of stroke care within their district and the provision of stroke care based on best practices and evidence.
- The DSC is accountable to adhere to the stroke line-by-line infrastructure allocated for stroke care for the provision of care and service. Stroke funding cannot be reallocated within the DSC's operating budget.
- The DSC is accountable to maintain and submit separate quarterly and year-end financial reports on the stroke infrastructure.
- The DSC will sustain the stroke infrastructure roles, descriptions, responsibilities and requirements as per Section B of the Service Guidelines.
- The DSC will work in partnership with their health-care community including District Health Councils, the rehabilitation and long-term care community, community acute hospitals and Community Care Access Centres.
- The DSCs will also partner with other stakeholders such as local boards of health and the Heart and Stroke Foundation to fulfil their accountability in the leadership, development, implementation and coordination of stroke care for their region.
- The OSS aligns with the DSCs operational and strategic plans.

**Responsibilities**

1. Regional/District and Community Leadership

- Develop a district plan for stroke care across the continuum, which builds upon the existing regional plan as per the RSSC.
- Partner with other RSCs and DSCs where appropriate to ensure the province-wide system based on best practices that builds on the expertise of the centres, provides for the sharing of tools and processes to decrease duplication and develops consistency of approaches.
- Develop plans and reports on the status of the regional stroke plan to the MOHLTC on a scheduled basis.
- Administers the district and regional strategy to maintain the regional network.

- Ensure timely communication to all stakeholders (e.g. MOHLTC, local communities).
- Ensure the implementation of the regional plan for stroke care based on best practices and continuous improvement.
- Implement acute stroke protocols (e.g. ambulance dispatch communication policies, paramedic hospital bypass protocols, community hospital triage and transport process including bypass with clustered hospitals without 24-hour CT scanning or which are missing other critical acute stroke care components).
- Facilitate outreach services to support enhanced consultation in rural and remote areas of the region.
- Organize and continuously upgrade stroke treatment in the district by adopting best practices based on a model of continuous learning and continuous improvement.
- Working in collaboration with their regional and provincial partners to ensure the collection and coordination of key data.
- Provide leadership in measuring and monitoring by working with other stakeholders to define further data needs, collect data, assess performance, evaluate outcomes and develop standards.
- Provide consultation and mentoring to other hospitals in the region to promote access to rt-PA and other interventions and organized stroke care.
- Development of human resource capacity plan in anticipation of staffing issues/shortages.

2. Provision of Patient Care and Services
*The DSC is to be fully operational to provide 24/7 access to rt-PA care with established acute care rapid response protocols by July 1, 2005.*

- On-staff Neurologists/stroke specialists organized to provide service with an established on-call schedule
- Access to a neurologist/stroke specialist within 15 minutes of patient's triage.
- CT scanner on site, with available technical staff to access scanner 24/7.
- Protocols and processes to support patients accessing CT scan within 1 hour of referral
- Radiologist/Neuroradiologist accessible 24/7 (may include teleradiology).

- Neurosurgery accessible through established processes within facility or with the RSC.
- Rapid emergency care accessible through established triage procedure.
- Clinical protocols established for all acute aspect of care from the ED to inpatient admission to discharge planning and case management.
- Dedicated clinical team of specialists in stroke care (e.g. RN, Physiotherapy, Occupational Therapy, Dietician, Social Work, and Speech language pathologist (SLP)). If human resource issues in the region preclude the hiring of staff (e.g. SLP) strategies must be in process to still provide access to that care.
- Provide coordinated services for all high-risk patients to allow for access to prevention programs, clinics, referrals and communication with primary care providers.
- Develop end implement care guidelines that enforce best practice standards that include transition of care management.

3. Systems

- Demonstrated clinical leadership, board and senior leadership commitment and track record of working collaboratively, establishing alliances and planning structures for the region.
- Partnership agreements and repatriation guidelines/agreements with DSCs, community hospitals and local facilities (e.g. Community Care Access Centres, Rehab. facilities, long-term care) to ensure appropriate and timely return of patients to their communities (cross border issues to be addressed).
- Develop transfer protocols (to include redirect) for community hospitals that do not have access to CT scanning.

*Section B: DSC Infrastructure*

**OSS District Stroke Coordinator**
*Requirements*

- Licensed member in good standing with a professional college and/or member of the RHPA.
- Minimum of 5 years' experience in clinical care with the following skills an asset:

- Strong consultative skills combined with clinical, institutional and community development knowledge;
- Leadership, interpersonal, communication and conflict resolution skills, with the ability to work both collaboratively and independently.

*Responsibilities*

- The DSC Coordinator will participate in the development and implementation of the stroke infrastructure within the DSC facility to support the regional strategy, e.g. transition management of patients, inpatient team development.
- The DSC Coordinator will administer the DSC stroke budget in co-operation with DSC processes/procedures and in partnership with the Regional Stroke Steering Committee and regional strategic plans.
- The DSC Coordinator will sustain the role and responsibilities of the DSC in co-operation with the Regional Steering Committee and the ministry.
- The DSC Coordinator will be the contact person for the ministry regional office and/or corporate offices.
- The DSC Coordinator will act as representative for the DSC and the Regional Steering Committee and appropriate sub-committees and/or working groups.
- The DSC Coordinator will administer the strategy within their district, including developing and implementing support systems to maintain the network activities.
- The DSC Coordinator will facilitate the management of the stroke care system to be organized in the various institutions and agencies across the continuum of care (e.g. acute care, rehabilitation and community).
- The DSC Coordinator will identify district specific needs for provider education and facilitate the regional education activities in conjunction with the Regional Education Coordinator.
- The DSC Coordinator will develop a local network of care providers and consumers across the stroke care continuum to define, develop and implement the local Stroke Strategy in partnership with the RSC.
- The DSC Coordinator will collaborate with other stakeholders to ensure that the province-wide system supports the sharing of tools and processes.

**On-Call Infrastructure**

- Neurologist and/or Stroke Specialist physicians On-Call Fees are provided to meet the designation criteria in your role as a DSC.
- The expectations for the on-call physician includes but are not limited to:
- 24/7 on-call for provision of specialized stroke care to patients.
- 15–30-minute arrival/contact to the patient from time of call for appropriate patients and protocols.
- Provision of clinical leadership.
- Consultation (e.g. telephone, telestroke) to other physicians and/or regional specialists.

# Appendix B: Semi-Structured Interview Guide—The Social Organization of Best Practice for Acute Stroke—An Institutional Ethnography

Please note that this guide only represents the main themes to be discussed with the participants and as such does not include the various probes that may also be used.

## Background Information/Warm-up

**Thank person for participating, go over consent and have them sign, explain process, how confidentiality and anonymity will be protected, etc.**

- It would be nice if you could let me know a little bit about yourself. How long have you been practicing neurology?
- What is your area of specialization?
- How many strokes do you treat in an average month?

## Practice: General

- Let me begin by asking you to describe for me your understanding of the usefulness of rt-PA? Probes: *How does it work?*
- Where did you obtain your information? Your training? Is this typical?

© The Author(s) 2020
F. Webster, *The Social Organization of Best Practice*,
https://doi.org/10.1007/978-3-030-43165-5

- Is it something you use often? Why/why not? When would you use it? When would you not use it?
- When did it first come into use? Do you know what led to that?
- Who, if anyone, should use it? Why/why not?
- What is needed to use it?

## Practice: Acute

- Can you take me through a typical case in which you used or were asked to use rt-PA?
- Can you take me through a typical case in which you were asked to administer rt-PA but chose not to?

## Cool-Down/Wrap-up Questions

- Is there anything else I haven't asked you about that you'd like to add?

# INDEX[1]

[1] Note: Page numbers followed by 'n' refer to notes.

© The Author(s) 2020
F. Webster, *The Social Organization of Best Practice*,
https://doi.org/10.1007/978-3-030-43165-5